PRAISE FOR *BLACKTHORN'S B*

"*Blackthorn's Botanical Magic* really reached inside my soul and chimed a ring of truth. Beautifully written, using contemporary magic to heighten and empower your life, I found it a wonderfully informative read, covering all manner of herbal witchery including essential oils and herbal plants to enlighten the reader. A must-have book for all those Green Witches, Kitchen Witches, and Hedge Witches out there!" —Leanna Greenaway, author of *Wicca Plain & Simple* and coauthor of *Wiccapedia*

"What a fresh new voice! *Blackthorn's Botanical Magic* has wisdom for the novice, the experienced herbalist, and everyone in between. Amy Blackthorn's style is accessible and the information so valuable in these anxiety-provoking times. Get this book and practice what you learn here." —H. Byron Ballard, author of *Earth Works: Ceremonies in Tower Time* and *Embracing Willendorf: A Witch's Way of Loving Your Body to Health and Fitness*

"Brilliantly written and jam-packed with practical advice and easy-to-follow recipes, *Blackthorn's Botanical Magic* is the one book that no magical practitioner can do without. I wish I'd had it when I began my practice!" —Dorothy Morrison, author of *Everyday Magic* and *The Craft*

"I absolutely love this book! Amy Blackthorn's vast experience with herbs and oils is evident on every page, and her friendly, wise, and witty voice makes it a pleasure to read. I particularly liked the chapter on using herbs in cleansing smoke, as well as the attention given to base oils and their various magical uses. The entries for each herb are rich with lore, recipes, and magical uses. This unique reference is a must-have for anyone who wants to get serious about using essential oils in their magic!" —Lisa Chamberlain, author of *Wicca Herbal Magic,* and host of *WiccaLiving.com*

"So much wisdom is packed into *Blackthorn's Botanical Magic*. The flow of information seamlessly blends the practical, scientific, historical, and magickal without overwhelming the reader, yet offering new ideas for a seasoned green witch." —Christopher Penczak, author and cofounder of the Temple of Witchcraft

"*Blackthorn's Botanical Magic* is a fantastic starter guide and takes such care in speaking about the origins and cultural connections of various plants and herbs. If you're looking for a practical guide that also takes time to answer how and why we're drawn to botanical magic, this is it." —Jaya Saxena, coauthor of *Basic Witches*

"*Blackthorn's Botanical Magic* is a valuable resource that fills the need for information about the magical properties of essential oils. A book unlike any other, it guides the reader through the world of essential oils describing their origins and dispelling the myths that surround them. The compendium of oils is a treasure trove of information, filled with magical correspondences, lore, therapeutic applications, and scores of original recipes for using oils, herbs, and other botanical ingredients for making magic. This book belongs in the library of every occultist, healer, and herbalist interested in incorporating essential oils into their practice." —Nicholas Pearson, author of *The Seven Archetypal Stones* and *Crystal Healing for the Heart*

"In her signature style, Amy Blackthorn offers botanical entries that are thorough and informative, with herbal lore to satisfy, and so many rich, inspired recipes for magical intentions—spells—all based on aromatherapy. Carrier oils are well-discussed as are ways to use magical essential oils every day. There are even recipes using other types of botanicals such as chili pepper and whole clove, which I consider a real bonus." —Doreen Shababy, author of *The Wild & Weedy Apothecary*

"If you haven't heard of Amy Blackthorn, well, you should. Not just because her tea (Blackthorn Hoodoo Blends) is delicious, let alone magical, but because Amy is an authority on herbs, oils, and brews of all sorts. I've witnessed her identify flowers in the field by name, species, and genus, detect the notes in the essential oil I was wearing, and whip up just the right concoction of herbs to go with pork chops.

Her formulas are efficacious and her knowledge of all things aromatherapy deep. She brings this expertise, as well as a charming, warm, and genuine voice to *Blackthorn's Botanical Magic*. Beginner or expert, magical or mundane . . . if you work with plants in any way, shape, or form, you need this book in your life." —Natalie Zaman, award-winning author of *Magical Destinations of the Northeast* and *Color and Conjure*

"To be a witch is to work with the powers of nature, and the green power of the plant kingdom is one of the greatest of all. *Blackthorn's Botanical Magic* is a resource for anyone who works with plant materials, whether they have just planted the first seed in their garden of knowledge or are surrounded by an encompassing grove of long experience. This book is more than a dry tome filled with facts and correspondences, it is rich with the sap and the fragrance of the author's love of this lore. The author's hand tends the reader as gracefully as they would their garden, and that is a gift." —Ivo Dominguez Jr., author of *Keys to Perception*

"An aroma can trigger memories, moods, and emotions. It plays on the most primal part of our brain. The essential oil of an herb is where all the good smell is and is the *essence* of any plant. In *Blackthorn's Botanical Magic*, Amy Blackthorn shows us how to utilize essential oils to effect magic. In addition to the magical applications of pure essential oils, synergies (essential oil blends), and base oils, she gives practical information such as safety precautions and shelf life. This book is a must-have for anyone who utilizes essential oils in their magic." —Deborah J. Martin, master herbalist and author of *A Green Witch's Cupboard* and *A Green Witch's Formulary*

"Knowledge is power when it comes to botanical magic and Amy Blackthorn has filled her book with scientific and magical information along with easy-to-follow formulas. *Blackthorn's Botanical Magic* is a great resource for anyone looking to put the potent power of plants behind their magic." —Adam Sartwell, cofounder of the Temple of Witchcraft and author of *Twenty-One Days of Reiki* and *The Blessing Cord*

BLACKTHORN'S
Botanical
Magic

· · · · · · · · · · · · · · · · · · ·

The Green Witch's Guide to Essential Oils
for Spellcraft, Ritual & Healing

Amy Blackthorn

WEISER
BOOKS

This edition first published in 2018 by Weiser Books, an imprint of
Red Wheel/Weiser, LLC
With offices at:
65 Parker Street, Suite 7
Newburyport, MA 01950
www.redwheelweiser.com

ISBN: 978-1-57863-630-3
Library of Congress Cataloging-in-Publication Data
Names: Blackthorn, Amy, 1981- author.
Title: Blackthorn's botanical magic : the green witch's guide to essential
oils for spellcraft, ritual, and healing / Amy Blackthorn.
Other titles: Botanical magic.
Description: Newburyport : Weiser Books, 2018. | Includes bibliographical
references and index.
Identifiers: LCCN 2018018499 | ISBN 9781578636303 (7 x 9 pbk : alk. paper)
Subjects: LCSH: Essences and essential oils--Miscellanea. | Magic. |
Witchcraft. | Nature--Miscellanea.
Classification: LCC BF1442.E77 B53 2018 | DDC 133.4/3--dc23
LC record available at *https://lccn.loc.gov/2018018499*

Cover and text design by Kathryn Sky-Peck
Typeset in Sabon

Printed in Canada
MAR
10 9 8 7 6 5 4

For Peep
(1947–2016)

. . . .

*[T]here is virtually no people known to
anthropology—however remote, isolated,
or primitive—which did not practise some
form of doctoring with plants . . . these
healing plants exert a beneficial effect on
every important part of the body, [and] may
have been carefully chosen to fortify . . .
man in his journey to another world.*

—Barbara Griggs, *Green Pharmacy*

. . . .

Contents

Introduction: No Magic Wand Needed!   1

1   Cleansing Smoke and Clearing Energies   7

2   Timing the Work   11

3   Making Oils Magical   15

4   Nine Myths of Essential Oils   37

5   Botanical Magic Starter Kit   41

6   Essential Oils from A to Z   49

7   Botanical Divination   279

Appendix A: Phototoxicity and Protecting Your Skin   296

Appendix B: Oils to Avoid During Pregnancy   297

Appendix C: Testing Your Essential Oils for Quality and Purity   298

Appendix D: Botanical Magic Resources   302

Glossary of Botanical Magic Terms   303

Recipe Index   311

Bibliography   317

Acknowledgments   321

No
Magic Wand
Needed!

Smell. That's right. Go ahead. Take a deep breath. I'll wait. If you are breathing, you are alive; and if you can smell, then you can enhance that life you're busy trying to live—no matter who you are.

This journey is yours for the taking, no magic wand needed! Aromatherapy and magic, one-stop shopping. Our sense of smell is the greatest sense, and even older than our sight. I'm Amy Blackthorn, witch, herbalist, martial artist, photographer, and your guide to the world of botanical magic.

Why botanical magic, you ask? Because by using our sense of smell, we can change our outlook, our mood, and even our dreams. What dreams would you like to fulfill?

People have been working with plants longer than we have had language. Whether or not you call yourself a witch; whether you have just purchased your first bottle of essential oil, or the local shop has you on speed dial; there is something in this book for you.

Before I get ahead of myself, though, let's make sure we're all on the same page.

What is this magic stuff, anyway? Rabbits and hats? No, my dear. Magic is agency. Magic is the ability to demand better from the universe because you damned well deserve it. Say it out loud. Who cares who hears you?

Magic is the ability to take all the feelings you have inside and turn them into something greater than the sum of their parts.

Do you want to banish womanizers? Do it.

Do you want to take back your power? Do it.

Do you want to reach far-off places, or just make sure you keep a roof over your head? Do it.

Magic can give you the sense of control you have wanted your entire life, no matter where or how you were raised. While we are forever colored by the things we have experienced, those things don't have to define who we are now if we don't want them to. The only person in control of the narrative of your life is you. Magic gives you the agency not just to change the story but to scrap the whole thing and start over if you want. Decide from moment one that you have taken control of your story, and you have. Magic is just the tool to help it along. You are the one holding the key. No magic wand needed.

I'm frequently asked how long I've been doing "this magic stuff." My first instinct is to reply, "How do you define magic?" For me, gardening is magic. Think about it: specks of dust go into the ground and beautiful things emerge from it. My first foray into gardening involved me helping neighbors and being paid in handfuls of loose change. I saved every bit of it, because more than anything I wanted plants of my very own.

I bought a green plastic window box and a bag of good soil that I lugged home on my bike without the luxury of a basket. I filled that window box with six packs of petunias, specifically Dreams Midnight Petunias. That was magic right there, boy howdy. Those flowers were a shade of purple so dark that the center of each one was black, and they smelled like the leading edge of a summer thunderstorm over a raging ocean. Magic was taking care of those fragile-looking stems and being rewarded with flowers that looked like velvet umbrellas filled with song.

In high school I chose to pursue a two-year botany and floriculture program instead of a traditional school experience. I had never been happier. I was already studying witchcraft by that point, and my love of herbalism, growing plants, and horticulture never faded. My independent study project was to grow all the herbs I wanted, all year. I bartered with the culinary students, trading herbs for free food (what high schooler would turn down Real Food?), and built up my own personal stores of herbs. I perfected my potions. The popular girls who would never admit to being curious about what I did came to me for the secrets of my clear skin and pleasant outlook. (For you, dear reader, my secret was weekly steam facials with rosemary and calendula.)

The secret to magic is stillness, being able to block out distractions, and letting go once the magic is in motion. Spells are directing the energies where we need them to go, through many methods (candles, singing, dancing, and more). In our society, we teach magic to children before they know their own names. We practice nearly worldwide sympathetic magic at least once a year.

Don't believe me? Think back to children's birthday parties. On their first birthday, before a child knows what a candle is, they're taught candle magic. Your nearest and dearest disappear and candles appear. The birthday song is sung, raising energy and setting the intention. The birthday boy or girl closes their eyes and makes a wish. They blow out the candle, cementing the intention. And then comes everyone's favorite part: cake. (Cake is scientifically proven to cause happiness. Eating after spell work also happens to be the quick and easy way to ground excess energy.)

PROCESS FOR CANDLE MAGIC:

1. *Decide on a goal.* One popular example would be money.

2. *Visualize the end result.* Maybe you need $42 to pay a parking ticket.

3. *Focus your intent to manifest that end result.* There are lots of ways to focus that intent. Maybe it's with a money chant. For example, I use The O'Jays song, "For the Love of Money." *Money, money money, money, MON-EY.*

4. *Light the candle.*

5. *Set it and forget it.* (Wait, that's an infomercial . . . forget I said that.) Seriously, though, if you obsess about the working, you're undoing all that hard work. Let the magic do its job.

Bonus tip: Make sure the candle you are using is "virgin." Don't use a candle that has already been used for another purpose, or you'll muddy the magic. One intention per candle only.

What is one of the few events that is celebrated nearly everywhere on the planet? New Year's Eve. And all over the world, people celebrate in their own way: tidying their homes, stocking larders and kitchens, spending time with friends and loved ones, counting down to midnight. What happens when the time comes? Kissing, cheering, hugging, joyous noise. Champagne toasts are traditional as well. Why? We are using sympathetic magic in an attempt to sweeten the year ahead. Sympathetic magic involves using symbols associated with an event or person to be influenced. On New Year's Day, traditional foods are prepared to bring prosperity, sweetness, a haleful home, and loving family and friends. By making sure we enter the new year in a good way, we are performing a ritual action to affect the rest of the year. People are doing magic all the time—they just never stop to think about it.

The day I moved into my first home, my mother spent a good deal of time lecturing me on how to move in. There were rules I had never known, because though I'd moved a lot as a child, I'd never been in charge of the moving. After painting and cleaning, the house gets cleansed. Magical cleansing involves energetic cleaning as well as physical. (For more on this, see chapter 1, Cleansing Smoke and Clearing Energies.) Then the home is blessed. Before any boxes are allowed to move into the new home, there is a procession: a loaf of bread so the occupants are always fed; a bottle of wine so there is always drink; a jar of salt so there is always prosperity; and a new broom, so as not to bring old issues from the last house into the new one. These sympathetic magical tools help ensure a happy and healthy home. Magic is alive and well in our culture, but no one calls it that. It's just what you do.

So, why essential oils? Simply put, essential oils are the soul of the plant, distilled into its finest point. You can't get the soul of a plant from a synthetic. Fragrance oils can smell nice, but smelling nice is not the soul of a plant. It is not the magic. It's just something that smells nice.

Botanical magic is different from what you might think it is. Yes, spells, magic, and witchcraft have a reputation for needing a lot of accoutrements, certainly. However, with botanical magic you are going right to the source. You are tapping directly into the realm of magic, into the heartbeat of the earth, and creating a change for yourself—change that you control. That change can be utilized by anyone—yogis, therapists, witches, accountants, nurses—just by adding your will, desire, and energy. The magic ingredient is you. Without you, these are just oils.

You can use plant material in spellwork rather than the essential oil, just as you can use a single note rather than a whole song. But just as a single note will never be the same as Led Zeppelin's "Ramble On," a single bud cannot hope to compare to a bottle of lavender essential oil.

You can do anything. It's the botanicals that lend that extra connection to the world. You know, that place outside, where it's too bright to see your phone screen, and there's weather. I'm hoping I can push you outside your comfort zone on this one. The plants are out there waiting for us to remember them.

Cleansing Smoke and Clearing Energies

1

egular use of cleansing smoke with a variety of materials is beneficial to an energetically healthy home. Too many folks rely solely on one cleaning method and one protection method. For example, many people enjoy the way white sage (*Salvia apiana*) smells, and though it is a good ally for clearing and cleansing space, it should not be your only ally.

Just as folklore says to turn your garments inside out if you think you've been bewitched, so too should your home's energy change. Changing the energetic signature of you, your home, and your loved ones makes it harder for anything nasty to recognize you. True curses and hexes are much rarer than one might be led to believe; they take training, dedication, and effort. That being said, jealousy has a power all its own, and it does not need training, materials, or much effort—only the green-eyed monster. The resentment that jealousy harbors can lead to bad luck, accidents, and worse. You will find many options for protections, cleansings, and the like throughout this book. See the Recipe Index for a full list.

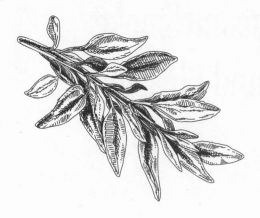

Sage is the go-to for many people, but you don't want to build the magical equivalent of a medically resistant staph infection. Change up your cleansing lineup on a regular basis. Maybe use Florida Water one month; anise protection incense the next; and then sweetgrass (*Anthoxanthum nitens*) after that. Then try burning frankincense. This is also beneficial in the case of witch wars and grudges. If friend X is no longer welcome in your home and they are likely to try bane work, having a varied protection routine makes it harder for someone to anticipate your plan of action and counter it.

SMOKE TOOLS

There is a hierarchy of smoke tools related to their efficacy.

The weakest of the smoke tools is floral smoke. Lavender buds, for example, are very pleasant smelling. Flowers are well suited to brightening a space.

Leaves are slightly stronger and are good for refreshing the energy of a space. White sage is a common example. Since white sage (*Salvia apiana*) is largely wildcrafted (harvested in the wild) and used by native peoples, the increasing use of herbal cleansing smoke has led to skyrocketing prices and difficulty in sourcing the materials for the native peoples to whom white sage is sacred. The *Salvia* genus has many allies that can be farmed and don't infringe on the beliefs and practices of First Nations and Native American people. There are many herbs found in this book that work just as magically.

The roots of a plant are stronger magically than its leaves. Roots will remove energies and entities that were not bothered by leaf smoke. Consider the strength of plant allies like ginger root, calamus root, and galangal root (Low John).

Even stronger than the root allies are wood allies. Palo santo is a popular wood-based smoke tool. This tree, native to Peru and the Yucatán Peninsula, has become increasingly popular in the last few years. This author even spotted it in a chain store that sells costumes, shot glasses, and T-shirts at the local mall. Because of the popularity of this wood, the trees that take decades to reach maturity are overharvested.

The strongest smoke tool of the plant ally families is the resin group. Tree resins are hardened sap structures like dragon's blood (*Dracaena draco*), frankincense (*Boswellia carteri*), copal (*Protium copal*), and myrrh (*Commiphora myrrha*). If there is a problem that has not been affected by the lower energy signatures of the plant allies, a resin should do the trick.

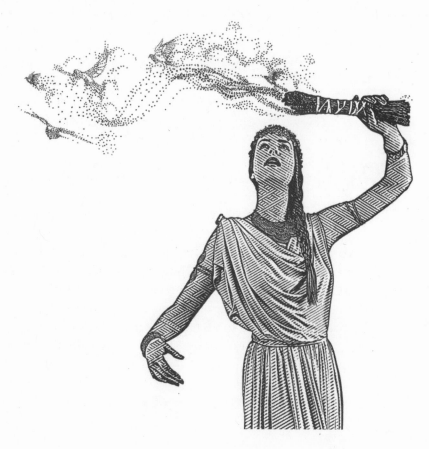

Dragon's Blood

This popular incense resin, resembling red chalk, commonly comes from two species, *Dracaena draco* and *Dracaena cinnabari*. Though there are more than the two varieties of Dracaena that produce this fragrant resin, many assume that all dragon's blood is *Dracaena draco*. Both produce a similarly colored sap, with musky, warm notes with a hint of floral, though *D. cinnabari* has a touch more of the floral note than its cousin *D. draco*. *D. cinnabari* is the slower growing of the two varieties, though both trees take over ten years to produce their signature red sap. Due to overharvesting and habitat loss, both species of Dracaena are on the threatened list.

Note: While no essential oil of dragon's blood exists at this time, high-quality dragon's blood oils can be sourced in Appendix D: Botanical Magic Resources.

Timing the Work 2

The timing of a magical working can make the difference in fighting against the tide and your magic making it to shore. Rather than putting extra effort to work against the moon or the day of the week, try rewording the working.

COLOR MAGIC

Essential oils are used in anointing oil blends, and candles are frequently anointed in botanical magic. Here's a cheat sheet of what all the different colored candles signify:

- Red—passion, fertility, enthusiasm, conquering fear, bravery, fast action

- Magenta—fuel for immediate action, enhances other colors, adds speed to magic

- Pink—gentle romance, friendship, honor, harmony, heart relationships, family

- Peach—quiet emotions of joy, strength, peace, truth

- Orange—adaptability, success, encouragement, uplifting, thoughtful

- Yellow—success, thought, will, intent

- Green—prosperity, fast money, healing past lives (use with brown for stable financial resources)

- Blue—spiritual and physical healing, wisdom, balance, trust, tranquility

- Purple—intuition, the Divine, guidance, power, ambition, prophetic dreams

- Black—banishing, hex breaking, breaking bad habits

- White—spiritual enlightenment, cancel magical aims, stalemate, purity, neutral (all-purpose), serenity

- Brown—stability, material wealth (physical goods, real estate), decision making, emotional balance, professional growth

- Gray—neutrality, can be used to cause confusion in an enemy if hexes are directed your way, self-defense, neutralizing harmful energies

- Gold—the God, fast luck, success, intelligence, solar influence

- Silver—the Goddess, resolve inner conflict, persistence, remove negativity

DAYS OF THE WEEK

Here are the best days of the week to perform each type of magic:

- Sunday—personal empowerment, success, generosity, luck

- Monday—spirituality, virtue, emotional security and well-being

- Tuesday—drive, confidence, ambition, victory, vitality

- Wednesday—knowledge, change, charm, communication

- Thursday—luck, power, protected growth, accomplishment, money, honor

- Friday—beauty, grace, the arts, love, fertility, bonding, sex appeal

- Saturday—the law, loss, endings, transforming, banishings, interrupting

MOON PHASES AND MAGIC

To give your magic a boost, try timing it with the phase of the moon. For things that won't wait, go with the day of the week that works best.

- Waxing moon—growing toward full. Do magic for increase, prosperity, health, wellness, love.

- Full moon—alignment of moon, earth, and sun (sometime resulting in an eclipse), all purpose, use the extra boost for the metaphysical heavy lifting, court cases, protection.

- Waning moon—shrinking toward the new moon. Practice magic of decrease; bringing things to a close; removing bad habits, negative people, debt, illness.

- New moon—first light. New growth, beginning projects, set ideas in motion. Set goals for the month.

- Dark moon—the absence of light. Do magic surrounding intuition, turning inward, cleansing, banishing or binding both people and addictions.

- Blue moon—the second full moon in a calendar month. Do magic for wishes.

- Black moon—the second new moon in a calendar month. Do magic for serious binding, banishing, stalkers, serious illness, addiction. Heavy lifting.

Identifying Moon Phases, Just by Looking

You may have seen a triple moon symbol; it looks like this)O(. It's not just a clever design; this is the waxing, full, and waning moon depicted. So, if you look up into the sky and the moon is pointing to the left, it is waxing. If it is pointing to the right, it is waning.

Making
Oils
Magical

3

To perform botanical magic, it's not necessary to memorize a bunch of recipes and formulas. Instead, my goal is to help you learn the basics, and then piece together blends for yourself to suit what you have on hand and what's happening at that moment. Eventually, you'll be able to stretch your wings and create your own blends.

ESSENTIAL OILS

Essential oils are present in more products than they are given credit for, and now, with internet-based retailers, boutique aromatherapy shops, and artisanal essential oils from farms, there is a surge in interest in the benefits of aromatherapy in everyday life. This includes magical practitioners. Knowing how these essential oils are derived is important, as it can affect the product's scent, whether you can apply it to your skin, and how much it costs. Let's go over some of the ways these oils are produced.

Extracting Essential Oils

Essential oils are single plants, broken down into their volatile constituents through distillation, solvents, or expression.

STEAM DISTILLATION

Steam distillation is the most common method of essential oil extraction and is used mostly for leaves and herbs. Here's how it works: Steam is forced up through a container of plant material into a condenser coil. The steam then collects and travels down the coil and drips into a specialized collection container. The liquid oil is lighter than water, so it rises to the top and drains off. The water left behind is referred to as a hydrosol.

HYDROSOLS

Hydrosols are the by-products of steam distillation that contain 0.02–0.03 percent dissolved particles of the essential oil that was created. They are scented naturally by the plant material they derive from. However, do not expect the hydrosol to smell exactly like its essential oil counterpart, due to the much smaller ratio of dissolved plant material inherent in the solution. Magically speaking, hydrosols have the same properties as the plant's essential oil at a lower price.

Until recently, many companies simply disposed of this beautiful water as a by-product of the oil-making process. But hydrosols are

Caveat Emptor

Experiment with different brands of essential oils whenever possible. Do not assume that just because an oil is more expensive that means it's more potent. An ethical company will clearly print on the label when they have diluted an oil, which is common for more rare or expensive oils. Commonly diluted oils include frankincense, blue chamomile, jasmine, melissa (also known as lemon balm), myrrh, neroli, and rose. Unscrupulous companies dilute other oils for their profit, so get to know the oils you want to use. For example, vetiver oil is dark and syrupy; so if the oil is clear and fluid, then either it's been diluted or it's not actually vetiver. (See Appendix C: Testing Your Essential Oils for Quality and Purity for methods of testing oil integrity at home with common household goods.)

valuable topical products in their own right. For example, one could use a lavender hydrosol as a spritz to call on the protective energies of lavender without needing to acquire and mix lavender essential oil, an oil carrier (more on this below), and mixing equipment.

Hydrosols are excellent bases for liquid smudge blends. They are gentle on the skin and can safely be added to the bath when an essential oil may be irritating. Many hydrosols are simply sold in pump bottles, as they make a nourishing mist for skin, fresh from the refrigerator on a hot day, or from the gym bag before you jump into the car to head home, and are sold as yoga mat sprays to freshen yoga mats after a vigorous practice.

Anytime a blend mentions water diffusers, it is possible to use a water-based room spray (or hydrosol) if a diffuser is impractical. Place 1 teaspoon table salt or witch hazel in a glass bowl and add 30 drops essential oil or synergy. Top with 2 tablespoons water and stir well. Transfer the synergy into a spray bottle and fill with warm water. Give it a good shake before spraying. Note: If essential oils are placed directly into water for spraying, they can leave oil stains on surfaces, so always use an intermediary.

WATER DISTILLATION

Water distillation is used for flowers that are too delicate for steam distillation. Water distillation can be accomplished at home with few materials and makes beautiful waters that can be used in magic, cosmetics, and aromatherapy.

SOLVENT EXTRACTION

Solvents are used to extract oils from delicate plant materials, namely flowers. The oil extracted with the solvent method is referred to as an absolute, such as rose absolute. Keep in mind the amount of time as well as the sheer quantity of flowers it takes to produce this material when looking at the price. For example, it takes about sixty roses to produce just one drop of rose absolute.

EXPRESSION/COLD PRESSING

Cold-pressed oils are a bit of a misnomer. The room temperature materials (citrus peels are the most common cold-pressed essential oils) are crushed between large rollers to release a dark-colored and highly fragrant oil.

SYNERGIES

A blend of two or more essential oils is known as a synergy. Synergies have a number of applications for our use. Ritual synergies can fill a room with a protective scent via a diffuser. Keep in mind that synergies have not been diluted, so they may be dangerous to put directly onto the skin. They are meant to be used in nasal inhalation tubes, room diffusers, or oil burners.

Caution: Please do not put undiluted essential oils on your skin without the direction of a certified aromatherapist. These are volatile oils and can cause chemical burns if caution is not used. Please seek the advice of a certified aromatherapist before using essential oils on anyone under twelve, and never use essential oils on infants. They simply do not have the body mass and will reach toxic levels very quickly. Although some vendors of essential oils are simultaneously trained professional aromatherapists, many, if not most, are not. Please be sure to consult with someone who has properly accredited training. Schools that train accredited aromatherapists will have listings that can be searched.

BASE AND CARRIER OILS

The terms "base oil" and "carrier oil" mean the same thing in terms of essential oils, and I use them interchangeably. Base oils can enhance the effect of your magic. The majority of base or carrier oils come from seeds or nuts. This is important for magic because the energy of new life contained within those oils can bring a powerful push of creation to any spell you use them in.

When choosing a carrier oil, consider the situation or occasion, the oil's shelf life, and your personal preference. For example, if an oil is being designed for a sabbat, choosing a carrier oil with a shelf life of three months means that a very small amount should be blended. Conversely, if the oil being designed is for a sabbat ritual attended by three hundred people, using an oil with a short shelf life is perfectly

Extending the Shelf Life of Oils

When creating oil blends, orifice reducers are important, not only to lessen the chance of a costly oil spill, but because the reducer will help keep your oils fresher, longer.

Adding a preservative to your oils can extend shelf life as well. Vitamin E capsules are a popular additive to combat oxidation, as is tincture of benzoin. To make tincture of benzoin, mix ¼ teaspoon ground or powdered benzoin and ¼ cup 100-proof vodka. Shake vigorously and let steep for six weeks. Vitamin E is a good preservative for massage oils.

Add 10 drops vitamin E per 8 fluid ounces of carrier oil, or 5 drops of benzoin tincture per ounce of carrier oil.

understandable, because many people will use the oil that day, and there will be very little remaining.

When creating an oil for your purposes, putting an expiration date on your label can save you time and energy. Properly cared for, your oil could last beyond the stated times. Trust your nose—you will know a rancid oil when you smell one.

Proper care of oil blends includes dark glass or dark number 1 plastic polyethylene terephthalate (PET) bottles, stored away from oil-destroying UV rays. A stable temperature is helpful, especially one on the cool side. Heat can be as detrimental as UV exposure. Oils with a short shelf life can be stored in the refrigerator to help lengthen their life span. Remember, even if they are kept out of light, oils are still susceptible to oxidation. This means that the longer the oil has been in the bottle, and the more oil has been used, the more space in the bottle that contains oxygen that can corrupt the oil inside.

Following are a few recommended carrier oils.

Apricot Kernel Oil

Apricot kernel oil has a nourishing effect on the skin, and its nutrients are easily absorbed. The penetrating action of the oil will deliver whatever has been added to it down into the deeper layers of skin, the subcutaneous tissue. It is well suited for sensitive or aging skin.

The benefit for magical practitioners is this oil becomes a part of you, rather than sitting on the surface of the skin with a greasy feel. The oil becomes part of the practitioner—a fitting visual for oils dedicated to certain deities and their dedicants. Apricot kernel oil is useful for anything related to Venus: love, the arts, beauty, luxury. It also works well in blends designed to facilitate a good night's sleep.

Apricot kernel oil's shelf life is six to twelve months.

Avocado Oil

On the skin, this oil is very penetrating and much heavier than apricot kernel oil. Cold-pressed avocado oil has incredible fats that make for a rich moisturizer for all skin types. It can help clear problem skin and has anti-inflammatory properties. It contains vitamin E and other antioxidants.

Avocado oil is magical by itself, and that magic involves creating new life and new beginnings as well as prosperity. That is just the energy of new life waiting to burst out of the seed. Because avocado has that round, full seed, it is useful in magic for fertility, including ritual oils for procreation, increasing sex drive in a partner, and lust. It's not just for physical fertility, mind you. If you need to make your business fertile, using an avocado-based oil is the way to go.

The oil of avocado has a relatively short shelf life, so make small batches, or only what will be used immediately. Use within three months.

Coconut Oil

Fractionated and expressed coconut oils are equally nourishing for the skin. The largest difference between the two is their room temperature states. Fractionated coconut is liquid at room temperature, while expressed coconut oil is solid with a low melting point. Many companies dilute their most expensive essential oils with jojoba or fractionated coconut oil to lessen the impact on the wallet. Coconut oil is a neutral-smelling body and cooking oil, and it is easy to find on the shelf in the grocery store. Additionally, it is easy to find organic coconut oil at reasonable prices.

Coconut oils are well suited to blends involving love, lunar magic, abundance, balance, childbirth or conception, good luck, or elemental magic.

The stability or shelf life of coconut oil is two or more years.

Evening Primrose Oil

Evening primrose is a very gentle, very light oil that is easily absorbed into the skin. It makes an empowering facial moisturizer especially well suited to the delicate skin around the eyes. Evening primrose oil is also highly regarded for its anti-inflammatory properties. Studies have suggested that it even has the ability to help children with hyperactive disorders and adults with autoimmune-related fatigue. (As always, discuss with your doctor before beginning any treatment, even with over-the-counter remedies.)

Using evening primrose oil in a magical practice has a.long history. This oil is popular across many genres and is thick enough that it is even sold as a drain opener. The plant's usefulness for wound healing means that it is connected magically with protection, boundaries, and sustaining luck. The "evening" portion of its name comes from the night blooming properties of this plant, which are associated with intuition, psychic ability,.and increasing vision. Evening primrose can be used to create egg shielding around your person.

Creating an Egg Shield

The visual of an egg is a popular one for establishing a protective shield around an individual. It is easy to erect, and maintain, an egg shield, and its blank canvas allows for later additions such as sigils (SIH-juls, magical symbols that translate to ideas). For a beginning practitioner, the idea is to spend time at first sitting quietly and picturing yourself surrounded by a strong, thick shell of an egg. (New practitioners have come back asking why their shielding isn't working, only to find that they have left holes in the shield for various reasons. That defeats the purpose, so we use the visual of the eggshell.) See that shell protecting you. Envision as much detail as possible.

Once the details are set, practice setting it faster and faster in subsequent sessions, until you can have it in place faster than you can blink. Remember, practice makes perfect! Some people put their shielding in place before leaving their home, just like putting on a jacket or sunglasses. Let your shielding protect you from magical threats as well as help you move through the mundane world.

Massaging the oil into the skin around the eyes before meditation, journeying, and channeling can help inner sight. For sufferers of night terrors, the light texture of this oil will lend itself to magical perfumes well. (See the Anise section for additional suggestions on combating night terrors.) Since evening primrose oil's shelf life is so short, it is ideal for long-term magical projects that are undertaken daily for one to three months—for example, creating a perfume blend for a devotional deity and applying it during prayer every day for ninety days.

The shelf life of evening primrose oil is three to six months.

Grapeseed Oil

Grapeseed oil has an ideal viscosity for skin applications. It has been known to hydrate skin, reduce wrinkles, and diminish the appearance of scars. It also has mild astringent properties, so it is useful for teenage skin or problem areas.

Since grapeseed is exceedingly good for skin balancing, why not use the oil for affirmations in magical practice? Anoint the tips of the fingers and massage into skin, repeating affirmations for the day:

I am worthy of love.

I am prosperous.

I am safe and whole.

Grapeseed's texture makes it an ideal anointing oil for oneself or deity statues. (Always patch test on an inconspicuous spot if you choose to use an oil on any painted or stained surface.) It is neutral and will not influence essential oils one way or another, so it is a good all-purpose oil for love potions and more. The long history of grapes and early civilizations makes it an ideal oil with which to announce your intent to the gods for a number of different goals. It's also affordable and easy to find in many grocery stores, making it a popular carrier for beginning oil enthusiasts and seasoned connoisseurs alike.

The shelf life of grapeseed oil is four to six months.

Jojoba Oil

Jojoba is referred to as an oil because of its viscosity, but it is not actually an oil at all. Jojoba is a vegetable wax that is liquid at room temperature. Highly moisturizing and good for all skin types, jojoba is penetrating and filled with antioxidants. It also has naturally occurring fungicidal properties, and so is beneficial for nail beds and feet.

Because jojoba is found in the desert, this interesting plant is used in magic involving perseverance. If something absolutely has to get done, jojoba is definitely the oil to go to for overcoming obstacles. Jojoba is used for overcoming the insurmountable and will not give up. It's also useful for oils based in self-confidence, as it is used to banish doubt. This oil also banishes melancholy.

Jojoba has a long shelf life, and though blends should be used within a year, it is not uncommon to see oil blends much older that have not yet gone rancid. Stability for jojoba is one to two years, depending on treatment.

Mineral Oil

Mineral oil is a petroleum distillate. The World Health Organization classified untreated mineral oil as a group one carcinogen, and it has been used to kill aphids and other pests. It is not recommended for use on skin.

Used in magic, this mineral oil is effective for any blend that involves minerals—especially if the recipe calls for things like sulfur or lodestone. Even before other oils can be added, mineral oil is beneficial for prosperity oils.

Mineral oil is good for oils of a compelling nature (getting someone to do something you need), such as the popular hoodoo oils like Boss Fix, Just Judge, and Bend Over oils. A recipe well suited to mineral oil would be "Binding Bending," found on pages 107–108. (For more information check out *BlackthornHoodooBlends.com*.) If you need something done right now, reach for mineral oil. It has been used by fire performers the world over, so use it for rapid change of circumstance.

Because mineral oil is not natural oil, but rather a by-product of gasoline production, it does not become rancid the way food- or seed-based oils do. If left for too long, however, mineral oil starts to gel, just as gasoline does. This gelatin-like consistency does not harm the efficacy of the oil, but with the prevalence of the oil, and the inexpensive nature of it, it is best to simply replace it.

Olive Oil

Olive oil can have a very strong smell, especially if you are not grabbing the more refined olive oils. Olive's soothing properties make it a boon in the bathroom as well as in the kitchen. Olive can help heal dry, cracked skin as well as skin with inflammatory problems. During the winter, keep a small bottle in the bathroom cabinet to massage into hands directly after a shower to lock in moisture.

This easy-to-use oil is usually on hand. When olive oil is used by itself, the effect of your magic is for blessings. It is sacred to a number of religious traditions, so it makes a good anointing oil. Olive oil is perfect for prosperity, as well as anything for good health. If you need hard and fast money right now, reach for this. If the goal of a spell has to do with tangible property, olive is the way to go. Olive is the friend of prosperity oils—but think "buying a house," not "I need $20 before payday." Folklore says that if a rich spouse is desired, olive is the oil to reach for.

Stability or shelf life is nine to twelve months.

Sunflower Oil

Sunflower is useful because of its affiliation with the sun. This is not just because it looks like the sun. This flower's big, fiery, orange-yellow brightness attracts all eyes in the meadow. The sunflower is the quickest producer of any oils.

What does that mean for magic? Prosperity. If you need quick cash, reach for the sunflower oil. If you need oil for the absolute best results, where failure is not an option, grab that sunflower oil. This oil is protected growth. For long-term goals—a year, five years, or ten years—you want to nurture that growth very slowly, and sunflower oil will shine its light upon you. Sunflower turns light into tangible food sources.

The shelf life for sunflower oil is twelve months.

Sweet Almond Oil

Sweet almond oil is commonly used in cosmetics and as a carrier oil in many different applications. It is very gentle on the skin and has a light texture. This oil is a good choice for massage oils, as it is not quickly absorbed, and anointing oils. Sweet almond is a nice alternative to the heavy feeling of olive oil.

In magic, the oil is useful for prosperity work. It is beneficial for asking the blessings of nature spirits such as the fae or daevas. The energy of sweet almond is that unconditional positive regard. Magically, it is a gentle oil and will work forgivingly. It is an all-purpose oil that is well suited for protection spells—especially spells involving children and their innocence. It has been used in love spells for that gentle, innocent first love.

The shelf stability of sweet almond oil is nine to twelve months.

Recommended Dilution

Here are some general rules of thumb for when you're mixing an essential oil with a carrier oil:

- 1 percent dilution or less: delicate skin areas, around the eyes and face; oils that are safe to use during pregnancy

- 1.5 percent dilution: emotional aromatherapy, energy work

- 2.5 percent dilution: massage therapy, general aromatherapy, skincare for thicker skin (elbows, feet)

The recipes in this book are calculated for 2.5 percent for skin safety and 0.5 percent with sensitizing oils like cinnamon. There are websites and smartphone apps that include dilution calculators. Above 2.5 percent is not recommended for magical aromatherapy. Discuss with a certified aromatherapist, massage therapist, or naturopath before using.

INFUSED OILS

Infused oils are made by placing herbal material into the chosen carrier oil and allowing the oil to take on the properties of the plant material over time. Let the mixture sit in a dark corner cabinet or

Tips for Crafting Infused Oils

- Dried material is always used to prevent molding.
- The key to infused oils is patience.
- With harder, woody plant material, the infused oil may not be ready to use for six to eight weeks.
- If you are making an oil for a special occasion, make sure to leave plenty of time.

··

on a shelf in a warm room for a few weeks. The oil will take on the properties of the plant material. Infused oils are much less fragrant than essential oils but can be used effectively in magic and may be significantly more cost-effective.

The benefit of making your own infused oils is that you can use plant materials that are rare, that are not available in essential oil form, or that are too sensitizing for cosmetic use but may be suitable for magical use. Plants that have no cosmetic or holistic usefulness can be infused to use year-round. The oils that are locked in the plant material will then be absorbed into the fatty oils of the carrier that is being used.

Many cooking oils employ this technique. For example, olive oil infused with Chinese hot peppers is frequently available at the grocery store. It carries properties of the Chinese hot pepper and is similarly useful for banishing spells.

This technique is also beneficial for plants that in essential oil form would be ill suited, too sensitizing for use on skin, or irritating in ritual baths. A practitioner could choose to break up several bay leaves and place them in a carrier oil to make an infused oil for communication, a protection bath oil, or a candle oil for love spells.

Purple dead nettle (*Lamium purpureum*) grows wild all over North America in poor soil and on the side of the road. This tempestuous "weed" (remember, "weed" just means a plant that grows where it is not intended to) is valuable for use in spells involving joy and happiness. While it has no smell, and is not suited to essential oil production, an infused oil is the perfect use for this herb. Simply dry plant material and add to a carrier oil. Dried plant material is more suited to infused oils, as water content can lead to reduced shelf life or spoiling concerns. For harder, heartier, or woody plant material, look to conditioned oils (see below).

Here's a basic recipe for an infused oil:

1. Fill a 4-ounce bottle halfway with carrier oil.

2. Place 2 tablespoons of dried plant material in the bottle and fill the rest of the way with carrier oil. Do not forget to leave room in the headspace for a dropper, if your bottle has one. Placing the herbs in the middle of the bottle makes the mixture easier to stir.

3. Shake the bottle daily for the first week, and let it sit for a minimum of six weeks before use.

Jojoba is a great choice for infused oils, as it is shelf stable for up to two years or more, when properly stored. You'll know if it goes rancid. Your nose will alert you. Rancid jojoba smells like burnt gym socks. If this should happen, just throw it away. There is no trick to save it. Dispose of it and get a new, fresh supply.

Here is a formula for vanilla-infused jojoba that serves as a love or gambling oil.

1. Slice a vanilla bean lengthways to expose the seeds inside.

2. Now place the two halves of the vanilla pod into a bottle containing jojoba oil.

3. Allow this to sit for several weeks. No need to remove the vanilla bean.

Looking for an uplifting infused oil to bring happiness?

1. Place a handful of dried orange peel into a clear glass bottle containing the carrier oil of your choice.

2. Let it gently warm in the sun for a day before moving it to a darker spot, such as a kitchen cabinet.

3. Store the oil for 4-6 weeks before use. No need to strain out the orange peel.

CONDITIONED OILS

Conditioned oils are similar to infused oils, with two key differences: the use of fresh plants and low heat. (The application of heat removes excess water from the mixture, so fresh plant material can be used.) Conditioned oils may have a stronger fragrance and a bit more energy than their infused counterparts. All that energy goes into your magical working.

With the advent of slow cookers and crockpot liners, creating personalized oils is much easier. Have the slow cooker on "keep warm" or low heat for conditioning oils, even overnight. The key is to keep the mixture at low heat because you don't want to damage the volatile oils in the plant material. Anytime there are plant materials present, make sure the lid is on tightly. After eight hours or so, turn off the heat and allow the oil to cool. Then bottle; no need to sit before use.

ANOINTING OILS

Anointing oils are popularly used for anointing candles, as well as people, ritual statuary, and more. This transforms the object or person into a holy one denoting reverence. Following are a few basic recipes.

All-Purpose Anointing Oil

This oil is beneficial for full moons, religious holidays, and any ritual or special day.

- 1 drop cedarwood essential oil (*Cedrus atlantica*)
  for consecration

- 1 drop clove essential oil (*Syzygium aromaticum*)
  to dispel negativity

- 2 drops frankincense essential oil (*Boswellia carteri*)
  for purification

- 2 tablespoons carrier oil

Reverence Oil

Anoint candles dedicated to the gods in thanks and ritual.

   1 drop cinnamon leaf essential oil (*Cinnamomum verum*)
      for uplifting

   1 drop ginger essential oil (*Zingiber officinale*) for healing

   1 drop pine essential oil (*Pinus sylvestris*) for cleansing

   2 drops sandalwood essential oil (*Santalum spicatum*)
      for calming

   2 tablespoons carrier oil

Goddess Blessing Oil

Anoint pulse points before meditation, prayer, or ritual.

   2 drops jasmine absolute (*Jasminum officinale*) for spiritual
      love

   1 drop peppermint essential oil (*Mentha piperita*)
      for consecration

   3 drops rose absolute (*Rosa damascena*) for harmony

   2 ¼ tablespoons carrier oil

Room Spray

Anytime a synergy recipe mentions water diffusers, it is possible to
use a water-based room spray (or a hydrosol) if a diffuser is impractical. Place a teaspoon of salt (table salt is fine for this application)
in a glass bowl, and add approximately 30 drops of essential oil or
synergy per ounce of water. Stir well. Once the oils are thoroughly
blended, transfer the salt into the spray bottle and fill with water
warm enough to dissolve the salt. Give it a good shake before spraying. The salt can be substituted with witch hazel from the pharmacy.
The essential oils need an intermediary because oil and water do not
mix. If essential oils are placed directly into water for spraying, it

can leave oil stains on surfaces, so use caution and always use an intermediary.

HYDROSOLS

Since these have a higher water content than their essential oil counterpart, don't expect a hydrosol to smell exactly like the oil. Magical practitioners need not do anything to it, as it has the same magical properties of the essential oil. It is much more affordable. Hydrosols are excellent bases for liquid clearing blends. They are gentle on the skin and can safely be added to the bath when an essential oil may be irritating.

Energy Cleansing Spritz

1 ounce juniper hydrosol (*Juniperus osteosperma)*
for protection

1 ounce peppermint hydrosol (*Mentha piperita*)
for purification

3 drops sandalwood essential oil (*Santalum album)*
for calming

1 teaspoon salt

To a 2-ounce spray bottle, add a teaspoon table salt, and add sandalwood essential oil. Mix well. Add hydrosols, leaving room for spray pump. Shake to mix. Spray anywhere the energy needs a lift.

BATH OILS

Cost-effective and naturally scented, bath oils are a major player in the list of oil tricks. They can be given as gifts at holidays and put together on the go after a stressful day.

Place 5 to 7 drops of essential oil into 1 ounce of carrier oil. This blend will nourish skin and leave you feeling soft and sweet-smelling. If there is a concern about slipping, consider mixing your essential oil into whole milk or powdered milk, rather than oil, and pour into the bathtub. The milk acts as an emulsifier, allowing the oil to mix with the bathwater. This makes a nice contrast to bath salts, which can have a drying effect on chapped or damaged skin.

BATH SALTS

Bath salts are a quick and easy method of dispersing essential oils into bathwater without the dangers of slipping and falling associated with bath oils. Magically, salt is purifying and beneficial for aching muscles and many other health and well-being challenges.

Basic Salt Scrub

Add 30 drops of the synergy of your choice to 2 cups salt and stir thoroughly. Pour desired amount under warm running bathwater.

If using a clear glass container for aesthetic purposes, mix small batches that will be used quickly. Store the excess salt mixture in an airtight container, preferably in a dark glass container or in a room without UV light exposure.

Note: Bath salts can have a drying effect on chapped or damaged skin, so consider using a bath oil in the winter.

SUGAR SCRUBS

Sugar scrubs can be enjoyed in the shower, but remember never to add sugar to bathwater. Sugar added to bathwater can feed yeast organisms and lead to an overgrowth, known as an infection.

Sugar scrubs vs. salt scrubs: Salt and sugar may look similar, but that's where the similarities end. When it comes to the types of skin on the body, the thicker skin (hands, arms, legs, feet) will benefit from a sugar scrub over a salt scrub. The salt scrub will feel softer on the face and will not have the sharp edges that sugar crystals do. On thinner facial skin, the edges of sugar crystals can lead to micro lacerations that can become infected and lead to scarring and premature aging.

Basic Sugar Scrub

4 tablespoons fractionated coconut oil (for a long shelf life)

2 gel caps vitamin E (natural preservative)

Optional: 10 drops essential oil

1 tablespoon honey

½ cup sugar

Grab a wide-mouthed, latch-topped jar. (Screw tops are difficult to operate when hands are slippery, and the grit can make getting the lid back on difficult.) Make sure the opening is big enough to comfortably accommodate your entire hand; it'll make scooping out the finished product easier.

Add the coconut oil to the jar, then pierce each vitamin E gel cap with a pin and squeeze the contents into the oil. Give it a quick stir to combine. If adding scent, add essential oils.

Add the honey and stir until incorporated.

Add the sugar slowly, stirring until completely blended. Add more coconut oil if needed until the desired consistency is reached.

CREATING AN ESSENTIAL OIL BLEND

While a book of this size can be overwhelming, it should be stated that no one is expected to memorize this much material before experimenting with magical aromatherapy. Each essential oil is structured to encourage a technique called "simpling." Pick an essential oil or three, and learn its every use. Use the oil(s) chosen for as many uses as possible, and really get to know them.

Think of this book as a dinner party, and each of the oils we're going to discuss as a guest. Having met "Petitgrain" once, it may be easy to remember that Petitgrain has two sisters, Bitter Orange and Neroli. However, if a few weeks pass without encountering Petitgrain, the names of her sisters may easily fall from the memory banks. Conversely, an encounter soon after meeting Petitgrain—three days later, for instance—will reinforce what you've learned about her.

By learning as many uses as possible for each oil chosen before moving on to the next, your memory will retain much more than if you read this book straight through cover to cover and then place it on a shelf. Remember, we retain a much higher percentage of what we learn by doing, rather than listening and reading.

Purchase the oils that smell the best to you (we are all pleasure-driven mammals, after all), and learn everything you can about them. The oils that smell the best will not only yield positive results but also a yearning to continue to learn more.

There are pages' worth of magical uses for a single essential oil listed. Once working with the oils chosen feels comfortable, it can be time to start branching out and trying the recipes. No one is saying buy four hundred dollars' worth of essential oils right off the bat. Start simple, and the lessons learned will stick.

There are useful recipes contained within this book, including an index of needs for inspiration. In the event inspiration strikes, or need necessitates, the instructions below are the steps followed to create each essential oil blend contained within these pages. Think of creating a magical blend as a Choose Your Own Adventure. Look down the line and see how things can play out before starting the blend to make sure it is exactly what is needed.

Step 1: Visualize a Need

Whether inspiration or necessity facilitates the creation of a magical blend matters not. The first step is to decide what is needed—the desired end result.

If the immediate need is money, the idea may need a bit more focus. How will that money be obtained? Money obtained painlessly is always the goal, but with rash actions there could be issues involved. If the goal is merely money, someone might convince themselves that a quick trip to the casino will solve the problem. The pain comes when all the money is gone and the problem is now worse than before. So a gambling oil is probably not the answer. However, if that someone has been loaning out money lately, it may be beneficial to call in some of that debt. Asking the friend to whom the money was lent is a direct way of handling it: "Hey, money is a little tight this month. Could you pay me back?" For some this could extend an uncomfortable situation.

Consider the alternative of leaving the money for the universe to dispense painlessly. That way it is not profiting from the death of a favored aunt, or a settlement from a disfiguring car accident. Forewarned is forearmed. Merely saying "money" can be too broad. Saying "I need seventy-five dollars, painlessly, to pay a red-light camera ticket (or whatever bill you may need paid) by next Thursday" is specific enough to be beneficial without constraining where the money has to come from.

Step 2: Make a List

Make a list of five to ten essential oils that can get you closer to reaching your goal.

If your goal is to get seventy-five dollars, you'd list all the prosperity oils, focusing on ones that bring good luck, attraction, drawing, blessing, manifesting, and removing blockages. The quick list will be citrus heavy, along with other scents that smell active, bright, and happy: angelica, ginger, melissa, neroli, orange, tangerine. Attempt to find a base note, a heart or middle note, and a top note that all fit the idea of prosperity, money, or abundance.

Step 3: Sample a Few Combinations

Once you've chosen three to five essential oils, take the lids off and place them on an index card in combinations of two or three. Smell different combinations to get an idea of how well the oils work together. If one of the oils stands out in a negative way, now is the time to replace it. Once oils start blending, there is no way to remove a discordant note—you can only attempt to drown it out with other oils. If the oils all blend well together, then it is time to proceed. In this example, May Chang, melissa, petitgrain, and vetiver were pulled from the shelf. Notice the strength of the vetiver oil in comparison to the other notes chosen.

Step 4: Record Each Chosen Oil's Associations

Once you've found a scent combination you like, write down the specific energies each oil brings to the synergy. For example, vetiver is a good luck oil, and a base note. It is derived from the root of the plant, so it will root the prosperity in the long term. Melissa (prosperity) and petitgrain (purification) are both warm, sweet, citrusy middle notes. They will lift the dark, earthy notes of vetiver. May Chang is used for strength, calm, and renewal, and has a sweet lemon scent that is brighter and sweeter than melissa.

Step 5: Blend the Oils

Every house needs a good foundation to stand on. The base note is the foundation for the oil and is the scent that will last the longest. Often base oils are heavier and thicker than their middle and top note counterparts. This will give the oil something to dissolve into later.

A 2 ml bottle can hold about 45 drops, depending on the size of the dropper or orifice reducers used. When experimenting with blending, it is best to start with a small number of drops and adjust accordingly. If the final oils chosen smelled harmonious, start with equal drops of each. In this instance, with vetiver being a bit stronger, this blend started off with 3 drops of vetiver, 6 drops each of petitgrain and melissa, and 1 drop of May Chang. May Chang is a very strong, very bright top note, so it was important to make sure it did not overpower the blend.

The bottle is capped, shaken, and allowed to rest for a few seconds before removing the lid and giving a test smell. A dot on a tissue may help to add oxygen to the blend to make sure it is performing as desired. If the blend is as intended, fill the bottle as much as is desired. With a rarely used need, it is less important to fill the container, especially if the blend contains expensive or hard-to-find materials. Once the bottle is filled to the desired level, make sure to replace the orifice reducer and cap to prevent future spills.

Step 6: Name Your Synergy

Now it is time to name your synergy. Fun names or self-explanatory— it's the dealer's choice. Just make sure to document everything. Recreating the blend is what takes magical happenstance and turns it into repeatable results, just like any scientific method.

Step 7: Review Your Work

Anytime you blend or use an oil, review the process. If the oil sits for a day or so and the smell changes, make a note. Perhaps the base oil used had not yet dissolved into the solution. If your intention for the oil did not go as planned, repeat the experiment. Several things can come into play. The oil could have performed differently than expected. The timing for the working could have been off. Or the work might not have been successful because it is not the work needed. A fellow teacher and dear friend H. Byron Ballard had this to say about a working she did that was not successful: "It wasn't my work to do. That wasn't my job." Sometimes, it just is not your work to do, and that is okay. (Seek out her work for amazing folklore, herbalism, and more.)

Step 8: Wash Your Hands

We're all adults, I know. But throwing out, composting, washing up, and everything in between each project keep the risk of contamination down, as well as the risk of chemical burns and phototoxic exposure. It also keeps our sense of smell intact. Essential oils are volatile chemicals. Safety first. As anyone who has touched their eyes too soon after cutting chili peppers can tell you, we don't always wash our hands as well as we think we do. (If you just cringed reading that, you know exactly what I'm talking about.)

Nine Myths of Essential Oils

4

hese myths largely drive sales, but can lead to dangerous misunderstandings about the nature of essential oils.

Myth 1: Essential Oils Never Expire

There are very few things in nature that do not expire. (Honey might be the only one.) Essential oils are a product of nature, and the leaves, fruit, and bark that these oils are derived from will eventually decompose. While essential oils may have a longer shelf life than their carrier counterparts, they will expire eventually. Here are a few tips to make your oils last as long as possible:

- Store oils in dark-colored glass bottles in a dark, cool place, out of direct sunlight. Light and heat can age essential oils.

- Keep lids tightly fastened—oxygen is the enemy of volatile oils.

- No matter how well the oils are treated, time will pass. Make sure there's a use-by date on each bottle. Note: Pine and citrus oils can irritate skin if used topically after their use-by date, even if they still smell good.

Expected shelf life for common oils:

- Coniferous and citrus essential oils: one to two years

- Herbal essential oils: three years

- Grass and resinous essential oils: six years

Myth 2: There's Only One Right Way / Oil

All-or-nothing thinking serves the essential oil companies more than the consumers of these products. If companies can convince buyers that essential oils can only be used for one purpose, this will drive them to seek more of their products.

Myth 3: You Need to Buy the Highest-Grade Essential Oils

There is no overseeing body that grades essential oils. The Food and Drug Administration has no hand in the essential oil industry because essential oils are neither a food nor a drug. Essential oils are not designed to be taken internally. There is no standardized grading system. There is no "Food Grade" or "Super Special Amazing Grade."

Myth 4: Rashes or Blisters Mean the Oil's Purging the Chemicals

No. A thousand times, no! Blistering is a sign of a chemical burn. "Chemical" is a buzzword used as a fear tactic to sell natural products. Reactions like this are a giant red flag. They can indicate an allergic reaction to the material making up the essential oil. They can indicate that the dilution percent is too strong for the skin it was exposed to. It could mean that the oil has gone bad. If you're having a bad reaction to an oil, discontinue use immediately and investigate the source.

Myth 5: Just Put the Oil on the Bottom of Your Feet

If the aim is for the body to absorb the essential oils, your feet are the worst place to apply. The skin of the feet is thick and callused, making it much more difficult for the oils to absorb into the skin. Ideally, essential oils should only be applied to the feet if they are specifically being treated, such as for pain or cramping.

Myth 6: There Is Only One Good Essential Oil Company

There are a lot of great essential oil companies. There is a difference between "We think we are the best company, and we hope you do too!" and "Every other company is evil and kills puppies!" Research and be willing to be flexible. (And see Appendix D: Botanical Magic Resources for a list of suggested suppliers of oils.)

Myth 7: Blends Are Better

Since this book details magical aromatherapy, we will look at the magical reasons one might choose to use a single oil:

1. *Developing a relationship.* Perhaps you are developing a relationship with a particular deity, and they are associated with a specific essential oil.

2. *Specificity in magic.* Using more than one oil can muddy the waters when it comes to the magic of choice. Each essential oil within this book is used in multiple magical blends.

3. *Cost.* Essential oils cost money, and not everyone has it to spend on a perfume organ's worth of oils. Hence the reason simpling is the best starting method.

Myth 8: Essential Oils Are Only Dangerous If Ingested

The myth about essential oils only being dangerous if they're consumed is alarming. Dermal application does carry risks. If used improperly, burns, rashes, and sensitivities can and do occur. Get trained. Listen to your body.

Myth 9: This Worked for My Sister's Cousin's Wife's Best Friend's Neighbor

Everyone is different. Talk to a trained professional. Simply because essential oils are derived from natural flowers, plants, and resins doesn't mean they don't have interactions with prescription and over-the-counter medications. (For more information, see *A-Z Guide to Drug-Herb-Vitamin Interactions* by Alan R. Gaby, MD.)

Myths drive sales; that is why companies benefit from sharing them. Do not allow myths to drive your health, hopes, or fears. Shine a light in the darkness for yourself and others.

Botanical Magic Starter Kit 5

n this section we'll cover everything you'll need to get started with botanical magic, in order of most important items to least important.

Essential Oils

If you are a beginner, your best bet is to get a few quality essential oils that can be used for a variety of applications. I'd recommend starting with the following oils because they have a variety of uses and are widely available:

- Bay (*Laurus nobilis*)

- Frankincense (*Boswellia carteri*)

- Myrrh (*Commiphora myrrha*)

- Lavender (*Lavandula angustifolia*)

Learn as much as possible about the plants you're using and add more to your collection as time and resources allow.

Assorted Bottles

Assorted small bottles are a must. This allows for small batch synergies, which save you money and reduce waste. Here are some common sizes you'll see throughout the book (see Appendix D: Botanical Magic Resources for a list of suggested bottle suppliers):

- 2 ml glass bottles or number 1 polyethylene terephthalate (PET) bottles (You will know it is PET because the universal recycling symbol, likely on the bottom, will have a number 1 inscribed in the center of the triangle.)

- 5 ml roller bottles

- 10 ml roller bottles

- 2-ounce spray bottles

- Orifice reducers (These are important not only to lessen the chance of a costly spill but also to keep your oils fresher longer.)

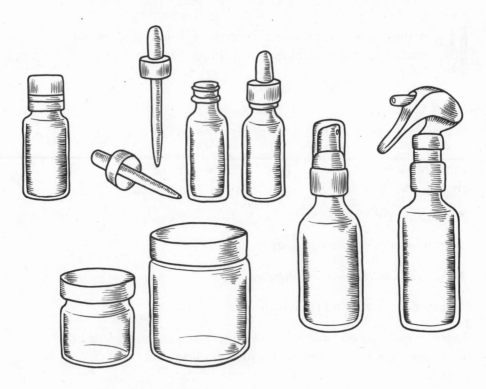

Vitamin E Capsules

Vitamin E is a good preservative for your massage oils. Add 10 drops per 8 fluid ounces of carrier oil.

Pipettes

Pipettes are a very important tool in aromatherapy. They look like long, thin eyedroppers and usually have a gradient on the side of the stem to measure liquid. Commonly they are sold in a 1-ounce size with gradients at 0.25, 0.5, 0.75, and 1 fluid ounce. They are primarily designed to be used once and recycled to keep from cross-contaminating oils. Depending on the viscosity—the thickness of the oil—an attempt can be made to wash a pipette, but it can be more hassle than it is worth.

Buy as many pipettes as is cost-effective and beneficial to do so. The reason for this is consistency of the size of the drop. Orifice reducers are helpful to keep oil from spilling, and they limit the amount of oxygen allowed into the bottle to a degree, but they are rarely uniform in size across different brands, and in the case of more viscous oils like vetiver it is easier to use a pipette to remove oil from the bottle than to wait for the drops to exit.

Stick Inhaler Tubes

Stick inhaler tubes are great. They have a similar size and shape to lip balm tubes, and when opened, there is a cotton swab shaped to fit inside the tube. This is also an important tool for those who work in scent-free environments such as offices, schools, and hospitals.

Labels

Labels are important and should include not only the bottle's contents but also an estimated expiration date based on the carrier oil and essential oils used. If the labels are paper, consider covering them in Scotch tape to preserve them, as direct contact with oil may cause the labels to fall off or become illegible.

Notebook

A notebook or note cards are a must. It would be nearly impossible to recreate an oil blend or perfume that worked well without having the notes behind it. If you're using index cards, try filing them in a recipe file box with A–Z dividers to stay organized.

Water or Salt Diffuser

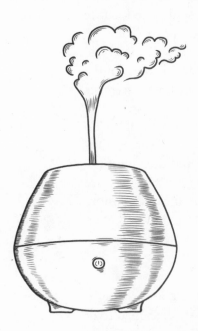

A water diffuser simply and effectively disperses essential oils into the air. It takes only one molecule of volatile oil for cells in the olfactory epithelium to detect an odor. Since these specialized cells are so important for survival, the body replaces them every thirty to sixty days, so they are always ready to go. A water diffuser atomizes the water contained within its reservoir and disperses it so much less of the essential oil is needed, thus saving money.

Salt diffusers are a no-energy way to diffuse synergies where a water diffuser is impractical (for example, around electrical wiring or electronics themselves). To make your own salt diffuser at home, add ¼ cup salt (table salt is cheapest, but large chunks of pink Himalayan salt can be beautifully decorative) to a large glass bowl. Add 10 to 15 drops of an essential oil or synergy of your choice. Place this type of diffuser in a cubicle where a pronounced fragrance might bother coworkers, or on a bedside table, where it can help you sleep without disturbing your partner. Because there is no water present, cleanup is easy and there is no danger of electrocution from electronics.

Tissues and Handkerchiefs

The importance of having tissues on hand cannot be overstated. Not only are they helpful for spot cleaning, but they serve many other uses as well. Place a drop or two of an essential oil or synergy on a tissue and gently inhale. This scented tissue can be carried in a pocket while running errands or otherwise away from stationary diffuser options.

Tissues are also valuable when blending essential oils into a synergy, as it can be difficult to judge the aroma of an oil. Simply place a drop of synergy onto the tissue and wave it under your nose to get a better idea of what the oils smell like when married in an oil.

Aroma Locket

An aroma locket is a pendant containing a small piece of cotton used to absorb a drop of oil. These are ideal when you are on the move.

Note

Use caution with jewelry marketed as "lava stone" aromatherapy jewelry. Lava beads suggest placing undiluted essential oil on them for the scent to be released throughout the day. This still puts neat or undiluted essential oils into contact with skin and should be avoided. Blisters, burns, hives, and rashes are likely to occur. Use only diluted essential oils in anything that directly contacts the skin.

Cloth

Cloth or another material for charm bags is handy to have in a witch's toolbox. Handkerchiefs, bandannas, and pillowcases that have outlived their usefulness can all be added to the fabric pile to be used for charm bags. The point here is not to have the best, neatest stitches; the point is that, once sealed inside, the magic can truly have a focus. Whether you're using a sewing machine, a needle and thread, or (in a pinch) a stapler, the point is to securely hold the bag together. Depending on the situation, the bag may not have to be sewn at all, if it can be securely tied shut.

Flash Paper

Stage magicians use flash paper for a burst of fire in the palm of the hand without heat, smoke, or ash. Small booklets of flash paper can be had for about $3 online and can also be found in many local magic supply shops. Simply write an intention or desire on a small piece of flash paper. Setting the intention by saying it out loud can be beneficial at first, but it isn't required if you feel it. Then simply touch the paper to a flame, and *whoosh*. A flash of light, without heat or smoke, and then nothing's left. All that heat will help send your intention out into the ether.

Wooden Box

Storage solutions are doubly important with aromatherapy materials. Oils should be stored in a dark place away from direct sunlight. Wooden boxes are ideal, as they insulate from light as well as drastic heat and cold that could prematurely age oils.

Bar Coasters

Bar coasters are highly useful. These handy (and often freely distributed) tools make great blending surfaces for oil creation, as they are so highly absorbent. They clean up spilled oils almost instantly, meaning a much smaller chance of irritation developing after accidental contact.

Coffee

Coffee is a nasal palette cleanser and is used to reset one's sense of smell. Smelling coffee beans can not only enhance the scent experience but also help train the nose to experience each scent. Both whole beans and ground are fine; just keep a lid on the coffee to preserve the scent.

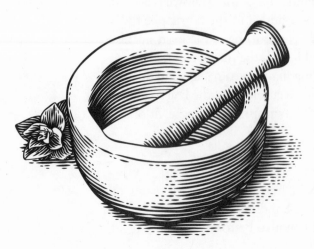

Mortar and Pestle or Coffee Grinder

A mortar and pestle is one of the most familiar stone tools from the logo of pharmacists the world over. Usually made from marble, granite, or another hard stone, it is used to grind herbs into smaller pieces or a fine powder. It's useful for making incense and charm bags, as well as mixing herbs of different textures for charms and spells. When searching for this valuable tool, don't be tempted by cheaper wooden versions; they are too soft to grind resins and will absorb oils, leading to rancid smells. Best to stay with stone or coffee grinders.

Stones

Stones can act as magical batteries. While specific stones are mentioned in the entry for each plant, there are a near infinite number of stones to choose from for the purpose of magic. To learn more about crystal magic, see *The Book of Stones* by Robert Simmons and Naisha Ahsian. And Melody's *Love Is in the Earth: A Kaleidoscope of Crystals (Updated)* is a comprehensive reference to the mineral kingdom, but the original volume does not include photos, so it is of more use to experienced practitioners who can identify the stones they are working with.

When using stones in charm bags, smaller is usually better. The stone's size will not impact its effect, and once the spell, working, or intention has been completed the charm can be opened and the stone removed, cleansed, and set aside to be used again. Simply compost or discard the materials as appropriate.

Essential Oils from A to Z

6

Before we jump in, I'd like to explain a bit about what the next section entails. Each plant in this section is referenced by its common name; this is the name we know the plant by in the spice aisle.

Scientific name: the Latin name(s)

Botanical family: important, because botanical families have similar actions and properties

Origin: where in the world the materials are largely sourced

Source of plant's oil: the part of the plant the essential oil is sourced from (e.g., roots, flowers, etc.)

Evaporation: whether it's a top, middle, or bottom note (the viscosity of the oil determines how quickly it is detected by the nose)

Scent description: features and notes of the fragrance

Scent impact: emotional effect of the oil

Magical Correspondences

Application: aromatherapeutic application

Element: of magic, earth, air, fire, water

Day: which day of the week best corresponds to magic worked with this oil

Magical uses: types of magic the oil is used for

Planet: the planet associated with the plant

Astrological sign(s): astrological sign(s) associated with the plant

Suggested crystal(s): stone(s) that could enhance magic done with this plant

Deity(ies)/spirit(s): helping spirits that could be petitioned for help, if desired

Warnings: specific cautions for each plant

Herbal lore: historical uses and stories about the plant

Uses: ways to use a single bottle of essential oil for magic

Recipes will have the featured essential oil at the top of the ingredient list so you can see the flexibility inherent in the magic of these oils. The rest of the essential oils will be listed alphabetically after that, with carriers listed last. For a list of recipes by need, see the Recipe Index in the back of the book.

Angelica

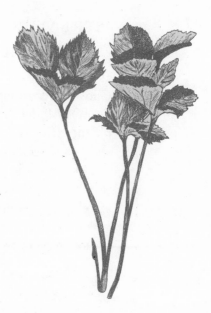

Scientific name: *Angelica archangelica*

Botanical family: Apiaceae

Origin: France, Belgium

Source of plant's oil: Roots, seeds

Evaporation: Middle note

Scent description: Earthy, sweet, musky

Scent impact: Releases negative emotions and thought patterns

Magical Correspondences

Application: Bath and massage oil, compress, direct inhalation

Element: Fire

Day: Sunday

Magical uses: Protection, grounding, lifting mood, banishing, healing

Planet: Sun

Astrological sign: Leo

Suggested crystals: Black tourmaline—ruled by Capricorn: grounding and protection; fire agate—ruled by Aries: spiritual strength

Deities/spirits: Archangel Michael—fire and protection; Venus—Roman goddess of love, sex, beauty, fertility

Warnings

Use caution if you are pregnant. Less is more with this oil; the scent can quickly become overpowering. Angelica is phototoxic, so avoid the sun for twelve to seventy-two hours after skin exposure. Try a patch test with diluted oil before applying the oil to a large surface area. Should be avoided by diabetics.

HERBAL LORE

It is suggested to grow angelica around your home to protect it, as one of the original epithets of the plant was "Root of the Holy Ghost." According to the herbalist Maud Grieve, author of the 1931 book *A Modern Herbal*, it was believed that angelica could cure the plague, after a monk saw it in a dream. It is said to protect from evil spirits and enchantment.

As indicated by its Latin binomial, angelica's heavenly connection has influenced its place in history for hundreds of years. Using angelica as a supposed cure for the plague was only the first step. It was dreamt as a cure for the plague by a monk who claimed he was given the plant by an angel. This supposed plague cure turned out to be correct, divine connection or no, because angelica has antibacterial properties. At the time, only two main areas remained unaffected by plague: Poland, because it gave asylum to the Jews, who had religious obligations toward bathing and therefore the bacterial growth had no grounds; and Milan, where if someone showed plague symptoms the house was burned down with the entire family inside.

> *If you have space for only one plant in the garden, plant the Angelica.*
>
> —Harald Tietze, *Herbal Teaology*

Angelica is said to have sprouted from the place where the Archangel Michael first set foot on Earth from the heavens. Thus, it has a long history of protection, both from evil spirits and more down-to-earth mishaps. It is so protective that some warn it can protect you from good opportunities as well as keep you from any harm that may befall you. Emotional shielding can keep out dangers as well as potential loved ones. Magical shielding can prevent beneficial energies as well as baneful ones. Protection should be encouraged and understood, without excess. There is an important line between protection and paranoia. Make sure that your interest in remaining safe does not guard you from beautiful experiences as well as horrifying ones.

Aromatherapists suggest using angelica in respiratory blends. The calming action and bronchial relationship make it a fantastic addition to meditation blends as well as protective oils and charms. Due to its affinity with the lungs and the characteristics of the notes, it will blend well with chamomile (sleep), lavender (peace), and lemon (healing).

Angelica is a strong, musky oil. Its strength, which comes from resin-like root material, makes angelica a natural fixative for any magical oil. The purpose of a fixative is to lengthen the scent's staying power and to act as a counterbalance to the top notes in a perfume. In most cases the top note is the scent you smell first. In the case of blends containing angelica, it is powerful enough to overpower the top notes. Angelica can also outlast some base notes.

Angelica is indicated for use in magical oils for those times when it is hard to believe in yourself. Remember, doubt is the killer of magical energy. If you doubt your spell or working will be effective, it is better not to do it, and come back to it later. You can take a walk to clear your head, talk to a magical friend about the working you are considering, or consult a divination tool. The magical friend is an important part, because it is hard to continue to understand where your doubts lie if all of your soul-searching reaps the return of cynicism or hostility toward magic.

Angelica can stimulate the mind, help release negative patterns in thinking, and clear feelings of emotional hollowness. This plant can also help you regain a connection to divinity, and is therefore good for use in dedication or initiation rituals or workings involving abundance.

USES

Place a drop of angelica essential oil on a square of tissue and tuck it inside your shoe when visiting a new open circle, or when petitioning to join a new coven or magical working group. It will help fight the "new kid" nerves that can crop up.

To attract good luck, place a drop of angelica oil at each outside corner of your home, or each interior corner if you live in an apartment, dorm, or shared space. Alternatively, fill your home with the scent by using an aromatherapy diffuser to gently waft a drop of this strong-smelling herb. This method will also help with purification of space in preparation for ritual and divination.

To prepare the body and mind for ritual, add a drop of angelica to your favorite shampoo or body wash. A few drops can be added to a salt bath for an adult to help ease grief, enter a meditative state, or reconnect with the gods.

Fill a custard cup with ¾ cup salt and 3 drops angelica oil. Stir with a popsicle stick or coffee stick to blend. Pour the mixture into a spray bottle and fill it with warm water. Shake to dissolve the salt. Spray around to protect the home, break jinxes and curses, or banish unquiet spirits.

To bind someone from doing evil, write the person's name on a piece of paper nine times, and take a pinch of angelica and a pinch of mandrake root and place them in the center of the paper. Bind it closed with twine or ribbon. Bury (or dispose of) the paper off your property.

Forgiveness Massage Oil

Heal a lovers' quarrel or learn to forgive yourself.

1 drop angelica essential oil (*Angelica archangelica*)
 to release negative feelings

5 drops German chamomile essential oil (*Matricaria recutita*)
 to dispel anger

3 drops rose geranium essential oil (*Pelargonium graveolens*)
 to release negative memories

8 drops lavender essential oil (*Lavandula angustifolia*)
 to balance emotions

3 drops lime essential oil (*Citrus latifolia*) to protect growth,
 increase strength, and raise your vibration

1.3 ounces jojoba oil

1 drop or 1 gel cap vitamin E

Mix all oils in a dark-colored glass or PET bottle.

For massage blends, a dilution of 2.5 percent is recommended (15 drops of synergy per ounce of carrier oil). Vitamin E is a good preservative for your massage oils, 10 drops per 8 fluid ounces of carrier oil.

Funeral Blessing Anointing Oil

This oil can be used to anoint the deceased's remains or to help ease the grief of loved ones.

1 drop angelica essential oil (*Angelica archangelica*)
    to recall pleasant times

1 drop clove essential oil (*Syzygium aromaticum*)
    to summmon courage

1 drop frankincense essential oil (*Boswellia carteri*)
    to lift spirits

1 drop myrrh essential oil (*Commiphora myrrha*)
    to promote spiritual awareness

1 drop sandalwood essential oil (*Santalum album*)
    to facilitate rest

4 teaspoons (20 ml) carrier oil

Fill your container with 2 teaspoons carrier oil, and then add the essential oils. Fill the container with remaining carrier oil, and put on the lid. Roll the container between your hands until the oils have been thoroughly mixed.

Home Cleansing Anointing Oil

Use this oil during home cleansing to bless the space.

1 drop angelica essential oil (*Angelica archangelica*) to protect

1 drop clove essential oil (*Syzygium aromaticum*)
   to bring luck into the home

2 drops sweet orange essential oil (*Citrus sinensis*)
   to bring prosperity

1 drop pine essential oil (*Pinus sylvestris*) for exorcism,
   protection

4 teaspoons (20 ml) carrier oil

Fill your container with 2 teaspoons carrier oil, and then add the essential oils. Fill the container with remaining carrier oil, and put on the lid. Roll the container between your hands until the oils have been thoroughly mixed.

Use this oil as part of a regular cleansing schedule—on the full or new moon is best. Sweep the home while chanting or singing. You may choose to carry incense or lit plant materials to each room in the home to chase away evil spirits. After you've finished sweeping, singing, chanting, then anoint the doors, windows, sinks (including garbage disposal, we do not want anything nasty getting in that way), and backs of mirrors (as they are also doorways into a home) with the oil. Once the ritual is complete, ring a bell and announce that the home is whole and protected.

Go, Baby, Go Anointing Oil

Get unstuck with this motivating oil.

1 drop angelica essential oil (*Angelica archangelica*)
   to exorcise

2 drops basil essential oil (*Ocimum basilicum*) to take flight
   (witches were once said to drink basil tea to expedite
   liftoff)

2 drops cedarwood essential oil (*Cedrus atlantica*) to increase
   focus

4 teaspoons (20 ml) carrier oil

Fill your container with 2 teaspoons carrier oil. Then add the essential oils. Fill the container with remaining carrier oil, and put on the lid. Roll the container between your hands until the oils have been thoroughly mixed.

Imbolc Oil

Use this blend on February 2 for rituals celebrating the Imbolc cross-quarter day.

1 drop angelica essential oil (*Angelica archangelica*)
   to sanctify

3 drops basil essential oil (*Ocimum basilicum*) to protect

1 drop bay laurel essential oil (*Laurus nobilis*) to purify

5 drops frankincense essential oil (*Boswellia carteri*)
   to consecrate

3 drops myrrh essential oil (*Commiphora myrrha*)
   to bless the oil

Combine all oils in a glass bottle. Add this synergy to a diffuser before ritual or add it to an anointing oil base.

   Note: Omit sensitizing bay laurel if this is going to be an anointing oil for the skin.

Blessings of the God Diffuser Oil

Diffuse this synergy when you need divine protection or blessings.

2 drops angelica essential oil (*Angelica archangelica*)
   to consecrate

2 drops cinnamon essential oil (*Cinnamomum zeylanicum*)
   to raise spiritual vibrations

6 drops frankincense essential oil (*Boswellia carteri*) for
   blessing, spirituality

4 drops rosemary essential oil (*Rosmarinus officinalis*) to
   protect

Combine all essential oils in a dark-colored glass vial (blue, amber, green) to block out UV light. Roll the sealed bottle gently between your hands to mix the oils. Diffuse one drop per 100 ml of water in a diffuser.

Hex-Removing Bath

Prepare this mix if you suspect misdeeds have been directed your way.

SYNERGY:

4 drops angelica essential oil (*Angelica archangelica*) to release
   negative feelings

8 drops clove essential oil (*Syzygium aromaticum*) to drive
   away hostile forces

8 drops ginger essential oil (*Zingiber officinale*) for success

10 drops lime essential oil (*Citrus latifolia*) for strength and
   to raise your vibration

10 drops vetiver essential oil (*Vetiveria zizanioides*) to
   overcome evil spells

BATH SALTS:

½ teaspoon synergy (about 50 drops)

2 cups Epsom salts

1 cup sea salt

¼ cup cornstarch

Optional: 4 drops food coloring

This blend has a very earthy scent for a reason: it is intended to ground the person taking the bath, as well as return any misdeeds to the earth to be transmuted. It is designed to harm none.

Mix all of the essential oils in a glass vial, and set the synergy aside. Then mix the bath salts. Pour the synergy into the bath salts, and stir to combine. Forty to 50 drops of synergy is ideal for this recipe, so feel free to add another drop or two of your favorite oil to this blend to make it your own. If it is pleasing to your nose, it will work better.

Blend well, and store in an airtight jar—preferably in dark glass, or clear glass kept away from sunlight. Use in a full bath, and visualize any curses or maledictions dissolving in the light of your radiant bath.

A Pleasing Odor

As you work your way through this book, you'll see that there are going to be some overlaps. One of the main reasons is that, in botanical magic, it is important that the end user find the blend pleasing. If they aren't comfortable with the scent, not only will they be reluctant to use it (it can't work if they won't use it) but the negative association can reinforce the negative feelings rather than the positive outcome.

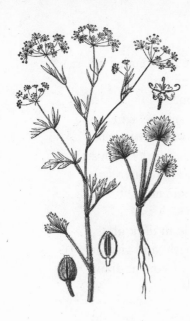

Anise (aka Aniseed)

Scientific name: *Pimpinella anisum*

Botanical family: Apiaceae

Origin: Turkey

Source of plant's oil: Seeds

Evaporation: Top note

Scent description: Sharp, piney

Scent impact: Release emotional blockages, helps recharge personal energy

Magical Correspondences

Application: Dilute, direct inhalation, diffuse

Element: Air

Days: Wednesday (Mercury), Thursday (Jupiter)

Magical uses: Love, fertility, purification, protection

Planets: Mercury, Jupiter

Astrological signs: Gemini, Pisces

Suggested crystals: Moonstone—ruled by Cancer, Libra, Scorpio: protection; rose quartz—ruled by Taurus, Libra; love, formed from the blood of Aphrodite

Deities/spirits: Apollo, Hermes, Mercury, Roman god of financial gain, commerce, communication (including divination), travelers, boundaries, luck, trickery, and thieves

Warnings

Use with caution if pregnant. Do not confuse aniseed (*Pimpinella anisum*) with its scent twin, anise hyssop (*Agastache foeniculum*), which can cause seizures.

HERBAL LORE

Anise is mentioned in the first authoritative book of medicines, *De Materia Medica*. This tome was the go-to source on medicine for over seventeen hundred years. One of the aromatherapeutic uses for this oil is to help combat arthritis, so using it in your magic to get unstuck is a great start. Whether you need motivation to finish a project or start a new life, anise can help you get motivated.

Perhaps its antirheumatic features explain its reputation of restoring lost youth. Books suggest hanging sprigs of anise over your bed at night or placing seeds in your shoes. For our needs, a drop of aniseed essential oil in each shoe will do the trick. If this does not help arthritis, at least we know the foot funk will abate.

USES

Place a drop of aniseed essential oil in the four corners of a space that will hold an open ritual to protect it from drama llamas, nasty folks, or just plain ennui.

If the energy in the home feels stagnant or murky, mix six drops of aniseed essential oil with baking soda and sprinkle around the carpeted areas. Wait an hour and vacuum.

Place aniseed in a pale blue mojo bag and place inside your pillowcase to protect against night terrors. In place of seeds, placing a tissue with a drop of aniseed essential oil inside the pillowcase will also suffice.

Anise has been added to wedding cakes since Roman times to ensure a long, happy marriage, filled with children. This is believed to be the origin of wedding cakes.

To make a difficult decision with the help of the gods, burn equal parts anise seeds and angelica root over incense charcoal.

Romans bathed in fresh anise leaves before marriage to protect the union and ensure happiness. You can also carry a sprig of anise to help you find happiness. Harness its power by adding a few drops of anise essential oil to a full tub of water or a drop into your shampoo before a date.

To protect babies from colic, place 2 teaspoons of aniseed into a blue pouch and hang near the crib.

For magic involving purifying the intestines or improving digestion, draw the outline of a person on paper and cut it out (think gingerbread man). Feel free to add squiggles where the intestines are. Add 1 teaspoon of aniseed or 1 drop of anise essential oil. Burn the paper and discard the ashes into moving water (a flushing toilet counts).

To reach other planes through divination, mix 3 drops of anise essential oil with 1 tablespoon of table salt and scatter it into a warm bath. Remember to bring a notepad and pen to record information received. Anise helps with sleep disorders, so try this in the evening for a great night's sleep.

For couples trying to conceive, place 1 drop of anise essential oil on a tissue and tuck it in a red drawstring pouch beneath the bed to encourage conception and boost fertility.

Psychic protection is another benefit of anise. Fill a purple drawstring bag with cotton balls and add 1 drop of anise essential oil inside. Carry it on your person.

Incense to Banish Evil

Burn this blend to clear a space of malevolent forces.

1 teaspoon angelica root

1 teaspoon aniseed

1 teaspoon whole or ground cloves

2 teaspoons ground dragon's blood

2 teaspoons myrrh

1 teaspoon black peppercorns

Incense charcoal

To banish evil forces from a space, mix all ingredients using a mortar and pestle. Burn the mixture over incense charcoal. Prayers to Hathor, the protective Egyptian goddess of joy and perfumery, are also helpful.

Divination Simmer Potpourri

Implore Jupiter to guide your hand with this mugwort simmer potpourri.

3 fresh mugwort leaves, minced, or 1 teaspoon dried mugwort

3 drops aniseed essential oil (*Pimpinella anisum*)

Place mugwort and aniseed essential oil in the glass bowl of an oil burner. Fill the bowl with water, and light a tea light beneath. This divination blend will help you discern the truth in a matter, make a difficult choice, or show you the way to happiness.

Joy Bath Salts

Sprinkle this blend in a bath to reclaim lost happiness.

9 drops aniseed essential oil (*Pimpinella anisum*) to help find fulfillment

15 drops bergamot essential oil (*Citrus bergamia*) for peace and happiness

6 drops rose geranium essential oil (*Pelargonium graveolens*) for protection and happiness

2 cups sea salt

Pour the essential oils over the sea salt and stir. Prayers to Euphrosyne, the Greek goddess of joy, as you draw your bath would be beneficial here.

Emotional Balance Oil

Use this oil to restore stability after a period of grief.

1 drop aniseed essential oil (*Pimpinella anisum*) to help find fulfillment

1 drop bay laurel essential oil (*Laurus nobilis*) for purification

2 drops heliotrope essential oil (*Heliotropium arborescens*) for optimism

1 drop rose geranium (*Pelargonium graveolens*) for blessing and happiness

4 teaspoons carrier oil

Add synergy to carrier oil and mix well. Ask for blessings of Maat or Vishnu, if desired.

Optional: Add a chip of moss agate to your anointing oil for added strength in all endeavors.

You can also blend these essential oils and add them to a nasal inhaler tube for on-the-go support.

Ritual Tool Consecration Oil

Use this oil to bless your tools and dedicate them to magical use.

1 drop aniseed essential oil (*Pimpinella anisum*) to protect and purify

2 drops basil essential oil (*Ocimum basilicum*) for consecration

2 drops patchouli essential oil (*Pogostemon patchouli*) for exorcism

4 teaspoons carrier oil

Optional: 1 small chip dragon's blood (*Dracaena draco*) to empower

Add synergy to carrier oil and mix well.

Anise Protection Incense

Smudge your home and loved ones with this blend to keep everyone safe.

Pinch aniseed (*Pimpinella anisum*) to move the negative out

Pinch angelica root (*Angelica archangelica*) to burn away anything nasty in the home or attached to loved ones

1 bay leaf, crumbled (*Laurus nobilis*) to create a circle of protection

Pinch of ground or whole cloves (*Syzygium aromaticacum*) to bring luck into the home

Incense charcoal

Blend the herbs using a mortar and pestle and burn over incense charcoal.

Depending on the size of the angelica root, it may be better to have an electric coffee grinder dedicated to incense use if you plan on enjoying incenses frequently. With just a few pulses you can have a consistent blend you can then burn over incense charcoal.

Night Terror Banishing Syrup

¼ teaspoon aniseed (*Pimpinella anisum*) for banishing nightmares, encouraging growth

2 teaspoons chamomile buds or 2 chamomile teabags (blend of *Matricaria recutita* and *Chamaemelum nobile*) for calming, psychic protection, dreams

2 cups sugar

Add aniseed, chamomile, sugar, and 2 cups water to a saucepan. Bring to a boil, stirring often. Boil two minutes and remove from heat. Allow to cool completely, then strain into a bottle. Administer 1 teaspoon before bed or after night terrors. Store excess in the refrigerator.

Psychic Protection Cookies

Believed to ward off evil, aniseed is the featured ingredient in these fragrant cookies. Ideal for sabbats and esbats.

DOUGH:

> 6 cups flour
>
> ¼ teaspoon salt
>
> 3 teaspoons baking powder
>
> 2 cups shortening
>
> 2 teaspoons aniseed
>
> 1½ cups white sugar
>
> 2 eggs
>
> ¼ cup brandy

TOPPING:

> ¼ cup white sugar
>
> 1 teaspoon ground cinnamon

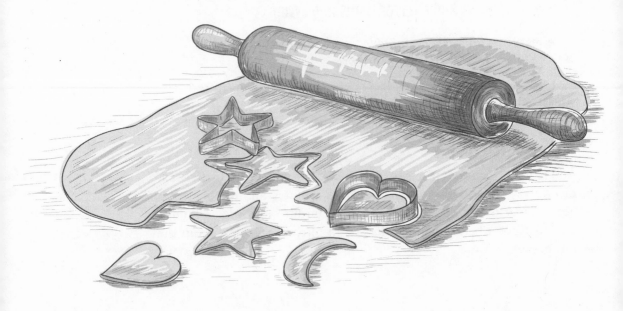

Preheat oven to 350 degrees Fahrenheit.

Sift flour, salt, and baking powder into a large bowl.

In a separate bowl, blend shortening and aniseed. Slowly mix the sugar into the shortening until fluffy. Add eggs, one at a time, and then the brandy. Incorporate the flour mixture, and stir until just combined.

Mix sugar and cinnamon in a small bowl and set aside.

Flour a cutting board and roll out the cookie dough until it's ½ inch thick. Cut out shapes using cookie cutters that are protective symbols, such as stars, and place cookies on a cookie sheet. Dust each cookie with the cinnamon-sugar mixture. Bake at 350 degrees Fahrenheit for 10 to 12 minutes or until lightly browned.

Basil, Sweet

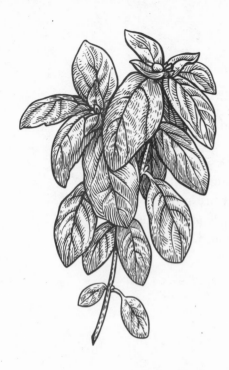

Scientific name: *Ocimum basilicum*

Botanical family: Lamiaceae

Origin: Egypt, India, France, United States

Source of plant's oil: Leaves, stems, flowers

Evaporation: Top note

Scent description: Light, spicy

Scent impact: Fight fatigue

Magical Correspondences

Application: Direct inhalation, dilute on skin

Element: Fire

Day: Tuesday

Magical uses: Love (sacred to Aphrodite), prosperity, exorcism, protection, memory

Planet: Mars

Astrological sign: Scorpio

Suggested crystal(s): marble, ruled by Cancer, helps develop deep meditative practice.

Deities/spirits: Vishnu, Hindu god, preserver and protector of the universe; Erzulie Freda, Vodou goddess of love and women

Warnings

Do not use sweet basil if you are epileptic.

HERBAL LORE

Basil has a recorded history of use in the culinary, magical, and medicinal disciplines, dating back over five thousand years, starting in India and working west to the Mediterranean. One of the most powerful stories relating to love and basil comes from Boccaccio's The Decameron. The story goes that Isabetta, a young lady with three rich brothers, fell in love with a man named Lorenzo who worked for her family. She started spending time with Lorenzo, and their love grew. When Isabetta's brothers discovered she had feelings for someone of a lower social class, they took Lorenzo out to the woods and killed him. When the brothers returned, they told Isabetta that Lorenzo had gone away on business. Though sad, she understood and retired to bed. That night, the ghost of Lorenzo appeared to Isabetta and told her where to find his body. The heartbroken Isabetta fled to the woods to dig up his body, armed only with a small knife.

Upon finding the body of her beloved, buried where his ghost had directed, she was inconsolable. She had fled so quickly, she had no means with which to retrieve his body for proper burial. In her grief, Isabetta cut off Lorenzo's head with her knife. She carried it under the cover of darkness to the family home, buried it in a pot topped with basil, and cried tears of grief. It was said that she cried so unceasingly her tears were used to water the basil and keep it alive. Sadly, her brothers discovered her grisly token and fled the city with it so there would be no proof of their evil deed. The poor Isabetta died of grief. To this day, basil is associated with lifting the sorrowful and supporting those in grief.

The relationship between basil and love became so strong that young men would place sprigs of basil in their hats if they had wedding bells in mind. Basil leaves were also considered a plausible test of virginity, fidelity, and companionship.

When visiting friends in a new home, bring them a potted basil plant; it will help ensure their home is filled with love, prosperity, and safety.

Uses

Place fresh-cut basil in a cup on your counter to keep it thriving until it is used in culinary dishes. The exorcism powers of basil will keep negative entities, spirits, and the like from your space.

Effective love spell: Place 9 basil seeds in a pot with soil. Water them, and tend them lovingly. Talk to them daily. Tell them about your day, the things that make you happy or sad. Tell the basil your hopes and dreams. This shows the varied goddesses of love that you are not only ready for love but have the time and energy to devote to a loving relationship. If you feel you do not have time to spend a few minutes a day talking to a plant, how will you find the time to devote to a loving relationship? This spell in no way impedes the free will of others; it signals to the gods that you are ready for a relationship and someone fitting for you will be placed in your path. It is up to the both of you to have a go at it.

Add 1 drop of basil essential oil to a room diffuser to help diffuse tension after an argument. It helps encourage both parties to talk and act with love in their hearts.

Add 3 drops of basil essential oil to a dark-colored bowl of water to increase psychic ability while water scrying.

During child blessing rituals such as wiccanings, use fresh basil leaves to sprinkle water on the child to bless them with love, protection, and prosperity.

Place a drop of basil essential oil on the bottom of each shoe to increase emotional balance when expecting a particularly trying day. It will clear a mental fog, improve focus, and decrease anxiety.

To turn aside evil: add a drop of sweet basil or holy basil (*Ocimum sanctum*) essential oil to 1 tablespoon olive oil and anoint the back of the neck and massage it into the bottoms of the feet.

Basil is associated with wealth and prosperity because it exorcises misfortune. Place a drop of basil essential oil on a photocopied one-dollar bill and place it inside your wallet or cash register(s) to bring good luck and prosperity to businesses.

To stoke the fires of lust between committed partners, place a drop of basil essential oil and a drop of cinnamon essential oil in a room diffuser.

Overcome sadness or sorrow by placing 1 drop of basil essential oil in 1 tablespoon of carrier oil. Dot on pulse points as needed. This blend lifts spirits, calms anxiety, and banishes melancholy.

Blend 3 drops of basil essential oil into jojoba or coconut oil and anoint all doors and windows in your house to keep evil from crossing the threshold. For best results, clean your home inside first to drive out any spirits that should not be there.

Ready for Love Anointing Oil

Use this oil to signal readiness for a new romantic partner.

　　1 drop basil essential oil (*Ocimum basilicum*) to draw love

　　2 drops tangerine essential oil (*Citrus reticulata*) for love and joy

　　1 drop patchouli essential oil (*Pogostemon cablin*) to arouse lust

　　1 drop lavender essential oil (*Lavandula angustifolia*) for love

　　2 tablespoons jojoba oil

Blend essential oils with carrier oil in a dark glass container. Anoint candles for love spells to signal readiness for love. Note: This spell will not remove the free will of others.

Alternatively, mix one drop of synergy per 100 ml water. Omit the jojoba oil.

New Addition Oil

Signal readiness for new baby in the family with this oil.

　　1 drop basil essential oil (*Ocimum basilicum*) for love and hope

　　2 drops rose geranium essential oil (*Pelargonium graveolens*) for fertility

　　2 drops sandalwood essential oil (*Santalum album*) for well wishes and healing

　　2 tablespoons jojoba oil

Blend all oils in a dark-colored glass container. Anoint candles to petition the gods for a new baby in the family.

Alternatively, add one drop of synergy per 100 ml water. Omit the jojoba oil.

Monetary Do-Over

Looking for a financial mulligan?

1 drop basil essential oil (*Ocimum basilicum*) for prosperity

1 drop bergamot essential oil (*Citrus bergamia*) for success

2 drops frankincense essential oil (*Boswellia carteri*) for purification

1 drop lavender essential oil (*Lavandula angustifolia*) for longevity

2 tablespoons jojoba oil

Blend all oils in a dark-colored glass container. Anoint candles to petition the gods for a new prosperous financial future.

Alternatively, mix one drop of synergy per 100 ml water. Omit the jojoba oil.

Burnout Biter

Diffuse this blend when nearing emotional exhaustion from witch wars.

1 drop basil essential oil (*Ocimum basilicum*) to increase sympathy between people

3 drops rosemary essential oil (*Rosmarinus officialis*) to cleanse and diminish the power of hurtful memories

1 drop vetiver essential oil (*Vetiveria zizaniodes*) for love

Blend all oils in a dark-colored glass container. Mix one drop of synergy per 100 ml water.

Focus-Pocus

Diffuse this blend when focus is of the utmost importance: ritual writing, initiations, dedications, elevations.

- 1 drop basil essential oil (*Ocimum basilicum*) to increase focus

- 2 drops ginger essential oil (*Zingiber officinale*) for stimulation

- 2 drops rosemary essential oil (*Rosmarinus officialis*) to improve mental powers, memory

Blend all oils in a dark-colored glass container. Mix one drop of synergy per 100 ml water.

Bay Laurel

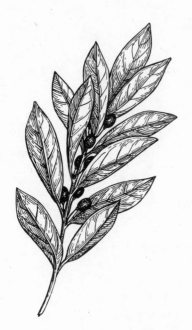

Scientific name: *Laurus nobilis*

Botanical family: Lauraceae

Origin: Mediterranean

Source of plant's oil: Leaves

Evaporation: Middle to top note

Scent description: Spicy, sweet

Scent impact: Boost self-confidence, lift mood, increase focus

Magical Correspondences

Application: Diffuse, direct inhalation

Element: Fire

Day: Sunday

Magical uses: Attraction, psychic talents, consecration, divination, good luck, hex breaking, love, protection, release, transformation

Planet: Sun

Astrological sign: Leo

Suggested crystals: Petrified wood—ruled by Leo: provides longevity in strength; Apache gold—ruled by Leo: intuition and awareness

Deities/spirits: Apollo, Greek god of oracles, medicine, knowledge; Daphne, Greek goddess of fresh water

Warnings

Use caution on damaged or sensitive skin. Never use undiluted on the body. Use with caution around children under five.

Herbal Lore

The list of uses for bay laurel, or simply bay, is considerable. The Latin binomial, *Laurus nobilis,* reflects the noble heritage of this shrub. Due to the custom of crowning Olympic victors in laurel wreaths, it has a reputation of overcoming obstacles of all kinds.

Mrs. Grieve mentions the use of bay leaves by the Delphic Oracle to achieve altered states of consciousness. However, excavations of the area have explained the oracle's trances through gasses leaching up through the ground in the antechamber, where the oracle composed her thoughts and prophesies. Still, the connection between the use of bay and psychic development and talents remains. No need to chew these sharp leaves, though; the energetic component of bay's abilities can be utilized in cooking (where a bay leaf or two can enhance the flavor of soups and stews), aromatherapy, and more.

> *And all the gods go with you!*
> *Upon your sword*
> *Sit laurel victory, and smooth success*
> *Be strew'd before your feet.*
>
> —Shakespeare, *"Antony and Cleopatra,"*
> Act I Scene III

An older common name for *Laurus nobilis* is Daphne, after the river nymph who lies at the root of bay's origin myth. The story goes that Daphne was adamant she would remain a virgin forever, so when Apollo came calling she wanted nothing to do with him. Although her father begged her for a son-in-law and grandchildren, she wished to remain free forever. When Apollo was not dissuaded by Daphne's wish to remain chaste, for he had been struck by Cupid's arrow, she fled. He chased her over mountains and through rivers, and when she was near collapse from exhaustion she cried out to Gaia to swallow her in the earth, and proclaimed that if her father the river had any power, he should change her rather than allow her to be taken as a bride. As she stumbled, her foot became rooted, her hair became leaves, her arms branches. As the bark covered her skin, Apollo proclaimed his love would never die, and he would wear the laurel as his symbol for all time; branches would forever be his crown and his temples would be filled with laurel. It is believed that Apollo's first temple was constructed entirely from laurel trees.

Readily available in garden centers, bay makes an attractive potted shrub and provides plenty of leaves for ritual, cooking, magic, and more. It has been a diner tradition for some years that if someone finds a bay leaf in their dish to wish upon it, for the wish would be invariably granted. The sturdy, evergreen leaves will keep for years to come. The bay leaves in your spice cabinet are perfectly suitable for magic. Just remember the spice rule: If they have color and scent, they're still viable. If they've bleached out all their color and no longer smell when crushed, to the compost pile for those poor souls.

Growing laurel has another benefit: brooms can be made of the branches. The laurel branch brooms were used to purify by sweeping a home after the death of a loved one. Saying prayers to Apollo while sweeping can safeguard the residents of the home. Laurel brooms were also used to sanctify holy spaces. If you are the crafty type, adding laurel branches to your ritual broom or creating a small whisk broom for your altar spaces would be a beneficial craft project. Online retailers have branches for sale, with or without leaves attached.

USES

Place three bay leaves, crushed, in a 15 ml dark glass bottle and fill with the carrier oil of your choice. Let it sit in a dark place for six weeks. Shake daily for the first week. This oil can be used to anoint candles for magic in any of the above-referenced intentions. The oil can be customized for any of the above uses by adding complementary stones or oils.

Use a drop of bay oil (infused or essential, your choice) on the bottom of each shoe when going in for a job interview. Remember, the victor is already crowned with laurels. Use the orifice reducer and cap to apply the drops onto shoes, as neat bay can make skin sensitive.

The communicative properties of bay are a favorite with teenagers. If you would like to hear from someone special, write their name on a bay leaf and put it with your phone, or even in your cell phone case. Magic is not a substitute for living in the real world, however. This is much harder to work if the intended does not have your phone number. Why not take the bull by the horns and give them your number? Everyone finds confidence attractive.

Is a friend going through a scary time, and you want to light a candle for them? Ring the candle in bay leaves to help protect them.

Want to dream of a future lover? Place three drops of bay oil on a piece of red flannel and place it in your pillowcase before sleep.

Use a bay leaf as a bookmark in your Book of Shadows to protect your sacred book.

Bay is also useful for commanding, banishing, magic, and enhancing magical abilities.

Obstacle-Removing Incense

Rid yourself of any lingering obstacles keeping you from your goal.

1 bay leaf, chopped (*Laurus nobilis*) to remove barriers to success

1 part frankincense (*Boswellia carteri*) to lift spirits

1 part myrrh (*Commiphora myrrha*) to calm fears about the future

Incense charcoal

Combine all herbs using a mortar and pestle or a coffee grinder dedicated to incense production. A finer grind will allow the bay to incorporate with the resin chunks more fully. Burn over incense charcoal.

Obstacle-Removing Diffuser Blend

Rid yourself of any lingering obstacles keeping you from your goal.

5 drops bay leaf essential oil (*Laurus nobilis*) to remove barriers to success

10 drops frankincense essential oil (*Boswellia carteri*) to lift spirits

4 drops myrrh essential oil (*Commiphora myrrha*) to calm fears about the future

Blend the synergy in a dark bottle and top with an orifice reducer. Cap, shake, and let sit if possible. To diffuse, add 1 drop per 100 ml water for small spaces. Think about your current situation (meditate if you already do so). See your obstacles dissolving while enjoying the spicy fragrance of this blend.

Happy Trails Oil

Diffuse this oil after breakups (romantic or platonic) to soothe yourself and gain closure.

> 7 drops bay essential oil (*Laurus nobilis*) for transformation and release
>
> 10 drops dragon's blood (*Dracaena draco*) for empowerment
>
> 5 drops rosemary essential oil (*Rosemarinus officialis*) to release and soothe memories
>
> 3 drops myrrh essential oil (*Commiphora myrrha*) to restore and lift mood
>
> 2 drops vetiver essential oil (*Vetiveria zizaniodes*) for strength, grounding

Combine all essential oils in a dark-colored 2 ml glass vial with an orifice reducer and cap to prevent spills. Shake, and add one drop per 100 ml water in a diffuser for a small room.

Note: As mentioned in the section on incense, there are many quality dragon's blood oils available, but a true essential oil is not on the market. For this recipe I used Black Phoenix Alchemy Lab's Dragon's Blood. For more information on sourcing oils, see Appendix D: Botanical Magic Resources.

All-Purpose Ritual Incense

Burn this blend before sabbat and esbat rituals to cleanse the space.

> 1 bay leaf, crushed (*Laurus nobilis*) to build a protective wall around the ritual space

1 piece cinnamon bark (*Cinnamomum zeylanicum*) for protection

3 frankincense tears (*Boswellia carteri*) for protection

1 piece myrrh (*Commiphora myrrha*) to lift spirits

1 teaspoon red sandalwood (*Pterocarpus santalinus*) to cleanse negativity

2 pinches blue vervain (*Verbena hastata*) for protection

This is a guideline recipe; adjust the amounts as needed for a pleasant-smelling blend. Protection blends work best when the scent is appealing to the subject of the protection. Always burn incenses containing cinnamon in a well-ventilated area so as not to irritate the lungs.

All-Purpose Ritual Diffuser Oil

1 drop bay leaf essential oil (*Laurus nobilis*) to build a protective wall around the ritual space

1 drop cinnamon essential oil (*Cinnamomum zeylanicum*) for protection

3 drops frankincense essential oil (*Boswellia carteri*) for protection

1 drop myrrh essential oil (*Commiphora myrrha*) to lift spirits

1 drop sandalwood essential oil (*Santalum album*) to cleanse negativity

Optional: 2 drops blue vervain–infused oil (*Verbena hastata*) for protection

Place all oils in a 2 ml bottle and use 1 drop in 100 ml water diffusers.

Long Night's Ritual Work

Got an all-nighter planned? Diffuse this blend.

- 1 drop bay leaf essential oil (*Laurus nobilis*) for increased focus
- 3 drops sweet orange essential oil (*Citrus sinensis*) to lift spirits and energize
- 1 drop vetiver essential oil (*Vetiveria zizanioides*) to enhance focus, uncrossing

Blend desired amount in a 2 ml bottle for use in room diffusers.

Doubt-Be-Gone Empowering Mist

Spritz this to remember how strong and capable you are.

- 1 drop bay leaf essential oil (*Laurus nobilis*) to empower
- 3 drops neroli essential oil (*Citrus aurantium var. amara*) to calm and bring joy
- 2 drops Brazilian rosewood essential oil (*Aniba rosaeodora*) to combat depression
- 1 teaspoon salt (your call: table, kosher, pink Himalayan, or another type)

Place essential oils into glass dish and stir. Add salt and mix well. Add to a small spray bottle with about 4 ounces (120 ml) water. Shake well. Mist over self. If needed, make muscles in the mirror until you laugh and remember that you are stronger than your physical body.

Note: Neroli is expensive. If cost is an issue, consider substituting petitgrain, which is derived from the same plant but distilled from the stems and leaves. It has a warm, green scent and a lower price point.

Bergamot

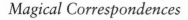

Scientific name: *Citrus bergamia*

Botanical family: Rutaceae

Origin: Italy, Ivory Coast

Source of plant's oil: Peels

Evaporation: Middle note

Scent description: High, citrusy, sweet, floral

Scent impact: Release negative emotions and thought patterns

Magical Correspondences

Application: Diffuse (see cautions for topical information)

Element: Fire

Day: Sunday

Magical uses: Manifestation, elevating mood, peace, success, prosperity

Planet: Sun

Astrological sign: Leo

Suggested crystal: Sunstone—ruled by Leo: dissipate stress and relieve anxiety

Deity/spirit: Ra, ancient Egyptian sun god

Warnings

Potentially phototoxic for twelve to seventy-two hours. Always dilute before use on skin. The furocoumarins like bergapten are responsible for the phototoxic reactions in citrus oils. Try to get bergapten-free (may be listed as FCF, or furocoumarin-free) bergamot essential oil for topical use whenever possible to remove potential for phototoxic reactions. Note: this will lessen some of the scent notes in the lemon family, so keep traditional bergamot oil on hand for diffusers. Old or oxidized oils can become harmful for topical use.

HERBAL LORE

Before we get down to brass tacks, it bears repeating that we are discussing *Citrus bergamia*—not *Monarda fistulosa*, or wild bergamot. The Monarda genus smells similar to *Citrus bergamia*, but do not let that fool you. They are not of the same order, family, genus, or species. This is one of the reasons scientific names are so important. These similar-smelling plants have different habitats, needs, and magical uses. I emphasize this because I found one magical herbal that listed *Citrus bergamia* but the illustration was *Monarda fistulosa*.

Wild bergamot has magical uses as well, but the two plants couldn't be more different. Whereas *Citrus bergamia* is a masculine, solar, and fiery plant used for success and commanding, *Monarda fistulosa* is a feminine, air-ruling plant benefiting mental clarity and bringing order from chaos. Both plants are available in essential oil form. For magical work such as this, make sure the plant being worked with fits the intention of the working first.

These differences are beneficial to magical aromatherapists. M. fistulosa ct. geraniol has a high geraniol content. This is what is known as a chemotype, a chemically different oil based on where the herb was grown, harvested, and extracted. The geraniol in this Monarda means it is antifungal and antibacterial, and has a cooling effect on the skin. Since it does not contain furocoumarins, M. fistulosa is not phototoxic. Blends can be engineered to smell like they contain bergamot without the potential burn of *Citrus bergamia* oil.

It is believed that bergamot was brought to Italy from the Canary Islands by Christopher Columbus. Bergamot was used in the very first recorded eau de cologne, and the scent is familiar to tea drinkers the world over due to its presence in Earl Grey.

The fruit of the bergamot plant is not eaten; rather, the peel is dried and used in tea, while the essential oil is used in perfumes, cosmetics, and holistic medicines. The use of bergamot in cosmetic applications is largely due to the fruit's ability to reduce fine lines and wrinkles as well as heal scar tissue.

Bergamot is used in commanding and compelling magic as well as blends for success, victory, and prosperity. It increases one's power and agency, and the ability to take control of one's circumstances. Bergamot is used to help accomplish one's goals.

Uses

Bossy? No, I'm the boss. Place a tissue with a drop of bergamot essential oil on it in a breast pocket of a jacket or close at hand when assertiveness is needed.

Anoint a candle with a drop of bergamot essential oil in a tablespoon of carrier oil for honoring ancestors.

Place 1 to 3 drops of bergamot essential oil on a tissue and place it in a pillowcase for restful sleep. This is also helpful for banishing nightmares.

Anoint a candle with a drop of bergamot essential oil in a tablespoon of carrier oil for spells involving joy and happiness.

Directly inhaling or diffusing a drop of bergamot essential oil in a diffuser can aid in concentration while studying (perhaps for a test from the High Priestess), or writing spells and rituals.

Psychic protection, on the double! Allow bergamot's fiery will to guard your third eye. Use a tissue or aroma locket to carry the protection with you without risk of phototoxic interactions—or dilute a bergapten-free bergamot essential oil in carrier oil and anoint the third eye.

Bergamot attracts desires well (especially physical objects), so write your desire on a sheet of paper. Then anoint a corner of the sheet and set under a candle (in a fireproof candleholder, of course!). Burn the candle to attract the desire to you. If you have it available, try flash paper if you intend to burn it afterward for a quick flash of light with no smoke, no ash, and no leftovers.

Time to Leave the Nest

Diffuse this blend to empower and encourage priests and priestesses with coven hiving, and bestow children leaving home with power and grace.

8 drops bergamot essential oil (*Citrus bergamia*) to lift spirits and encourage happiness, success

3 drops Texas cedarwood essential oil (*Juniperus mexicana*) for self-control and benevolent power

1 drop vetiver essential oil (*Vetiveria zizanioides*) for protection

6 drops ylang-ylang essential oil (*Cananga odorata*) for peace and successful ventures

Blend all oils in a dark-colored glass container. Mix one drop of synergy per 100 ml water.

Business Plan Booster

Magical folks hustle. Diffuse this to ensure success in business-planning magic.

10 drops bergamot essential oil (*Citrus bergamia*) for business success, hope

2 drops ginger essential oil (*Zingiber officinale*) for courage and money

2 drops rosemary essential oil (*Rosemarinus officialis*) for mental energy and protection

3 drops ylang-ylang essential oil (*Cananga odorata*) for successful ventures

Blend all oils in a dark-colored glass container. Carefully wash hands after oil creation to avoid phototoxic burns.

If you would like to add this to business success candle magic, add 1 drop of synergy to 1 tablespoon carrier oil and anoint candle.

Hypnos Hibernation

Sleep and the realm of dreams await, with the help of the Greek god of rest. Diffuse this blend an hour before bed to have magical sleep and calming dreams.

10 drops bergamot essential oil (*Citrus bergamia*) for peace, quiet happiness

5 drops Roman chamomile essential oil (*Chamaemelum nobile*) for sleep, purification, stress relief

7 drops patchouli essential oil (*Pogostemon cablin*) for grounding, physical energy

Blend all oils in a dark-colored glass container. Mix one drop of synergy per 100 ml water.

Best if enjoyed with a caffeine-free tea and quiet reflection. Avoid using cell phones or tablets before bed, as the screen lights can disturb sleep cycles.

Buzz Off

Use this blend to drive away unwanted persons.

15 drops bergamot essential oil (*Citrus bergamia*) to command power

15 drops black pepper essential oil (*Piper nigrum*) to drive away evil

5 drops clove essential oil (*Syzygium aromaticum*) for dispelling, hex breaking

Whether it's a former lover, a friend who turned out not to be, or a family member we wish would lose our number, there are always people we want to stay gone. Mix all essential oils and dilute one drop of synergy in a 2 ml bottle of the carrier of choice. Anoint a black candle for banishing on a Saturday (endings) to get someone to leave you alone for good. If the moon is waning or dark, all the better.

Here's to Success Cocktail

An adult beverage to celebrate and ensure success in endeavors mundane and magical.

1 wedge Meyer lemon (or regular lemon if Meyer isn't available)

1 tablespoon brown sugar

1.5 ounces Earl Grey–infused gin (see below)

1.5 ounces fresh lemon juice

2 ounces lavender syrup (see below) or simple syrup

Rim two martini glasses with the lemon wedge. Pour brown sugar onto a shallow plate and coat the rim of each glass. Set glasses aside.

Add gin, lemon juice, and lavender syrup to an iced cocktail shaker (metal is preferred). Shake vigorously until frost appears on the outside of the shaker. Strain into rimmed martini glasses.

EARL GREY–INFUSED GIN

Add ¼ to ⅓ cup Earl Grey leaves (it's best if bergamot is present rather than bergamot flavoring; try Earl Grey green tea for a brighter citrus burst)

1 liter gin of your choice

Pour gin over Earl Grey in a large pitcher and set aside for 2 to 3 hours. Strain the liquid back into the gin bottle with a coffee filter placed in a funnel. Resist the urge to wring the leaves into the gin, as it will make the gin bitter.

LAVENDER SYRUP

2 teaspoons lavender buds

2 cups sugar

2 cups water

Add lavender, sugar, and water to a saucepan. Bring to a boil, stirring often. Boil two minutes and remove from heat. Allow to cool completely and strain flowers out before bottling. Store any remaining syrup in the refrigerator.

Use lavender syrup in place of simple syrup for any beverage—coffee, tea, lemonade, etc.

Any sugar recipe can be made into a lavender recipe: simply add 1 teaspoon lavender buds per 1 cup sugar. Sugar cookies become lavender sugar cookies. Lemonade becomes lavender lemonade. Try lavender simple syrup, a lavender butter cake, or lavender brownies, just to name a few.

Black Pepper

Scientific name: *Piper nigrum*

Botanical family: Piperaceae

Origin: India, Egypt, Madagascar, Sri Lanka, China, Indonesia

Source of plant's oil: Berries

Evaporation: Middle note

Scent description: Warm, spicy, strong, herbal

Scent impact: Empower yourself and others

Magical Correspondences

Application: Diffuse, direct inhalation, dilute

Element: Fire

Day: Tuesday

Magical uses: Clarity of mind, strength, courage, clarity of purpose, alertness/perception, protection, banishing

Planet: Mars

Astrological sign: Aries

Suggested crystal: Sunstone—ruled by Leo: burns away blockages in chakras

Deities/spirits: The Morrigan, Celtic goddess of war, strength, and courage; Hecate, Greek goddess of magic, protection against hexes

Warnings

Keep out of reach of children. May irritate eyes, ears, or sensitive skin. Use sparingly, as overuse can cause kidney damage. Never consume essential oils without the supervision of a trained, certified herbalist or aromatherapist.

Herbal Lore

It is an herb with one of the oldest known traditions. Black pepper-corns were used in the mummification of Ramesses II. One of the spices that was exotic enough to have been used as currency, at one time as valuable as silver and gold. Trade routes were established between countries just to get the precious spice. When Attila and the Goths were sacking Rome, among their ransom demands was three thousand pounds of peppercorns.

Black pepper, an ally of law, justice, and strength, can be successfully used by those in the military, law enforcement, and the judicial system. This essential oil not only acts as a protective herb but also empowers the user through feelings of strength and courage. Use this oil anytime feelings of helplessness, hopelessness, or lack of agency plague you or loved ones. The strength provided by black pepper is not just emotional, though. It also helps uncover reserves of physical strength previously unheard of. Monks in India ate whole black pep-percorns to power their long journeys to prevent fatigue. The oil is physically stimulating, even increasing metabolism.

Use these stimulating properties if you need to stimulate income. The mentally stimulating traits also encourage business plans, ideas in general, clear thinking, and eloquence. Just make sure to back up all that stimulation with more plans and actions or the benefits will burn out quickly. Because this is an aggressive-smelling oil, other strong, stimulating oils such as clove, juniper, lemon, and lime will pair well scent-wise.

Uses

Place a drop of black pepper in a jar of black salt to increase its protective qualities and banish evil and spirits.

Black pepper is stimulating; place a drop on a tissue inside a pillowcase to spark the dreaming mind.

Mental stimulation works in the daytime as well. Put a drop on a tissue, in a breast pocket, if you have to appear in court to speak clearly, with thought and eloquence. For an extra boost, dilute

> ## Multipurpose Black Pepper Oil
>
> For sensitizing oils like black pepper, place a drop of essential oil in a 10 ml roller and fill it with jojoba or fractionated coconut oil. Replace the roller cap and lid, and give it a shake. Use the oil to draw sigils, or anoint candles, mojo bags, charms, and talismans without actually having to touch the oil to your skin. Just make sure to label it carefully.

peppercorns heavily in evening primrose oil (*Oenothera biennis*), as it helps remove doubt. This charm also works well for defending a thesis, presenting proposals involving business loans, and performing other public speaking obligations. It will help that anxiety-related nausea as well.

Place a drop of black pepper essential oil on the bottom of each shoe to turn aside evil and keep it from following you home. This is especially useful for paranormal investigators.

For tests of endurance, dilute a drop of black pepper essential oil in a teaspoon of carrier oil and anoint the heels of your shoes.

To banish an unwanted person, write their name on a piece of paper and, if desired, what they've done. Anoint it with 3 drops of diluted black pepper essential oil. (Wash your hands immediately if you get it on you, as it can irritate skin.) Anoint a black candle with diluted black pepper oil. Place the paper under the candle and light the candle. The person will vanish from your life.

If you choose to burn the paper after the candle has burned out, dump the ashes into a swiftly moving body of water and dispose of the candle remains off your property. (Ideal places include trashcans in large commercial areas, big-box stores' trash. Big-box stores and outdoor shopping centers are the crossroads of our modern society. The trash is emptied daily, and their turnover in product and foot traffic guarantees that even if you go back the next day it is a different store. It has different employees, different customers, and different goods.)

If the person you are wishing to banish has broken the law, dispose of the candle remains in a trashcan on the property of a courthouse. Boost the justice aspect of this banishing spell by incorporating soil from a courthouse. A small handful from the landscaping will do nicely and is easy to obtain. Place a pinch of the soil in the candle-holder, or place the target's name paper in a small container filled with the soil from the courthouse. Burn the candle as above. Throw away any remains from the ritual in the trash outside the courthouse.

Song of the New Wood Initiation Oil

Use for initiation rituals, oaths, new jobs, and when starting important projects.

  10 drops black pepper essential oil (*Piper nigrum*) to banish negativity, protect, and provide courage

  9 drops Texas cedarwood essential oil (*Juniperus mexicana*) for healing, purification, protection

  20 drops grapefruit essential oil (*Citrus paradisi*) for purity, mental clarity, initiation

  20 drops sweet orange essential oil (*Citrus sinensis*) for love, luck

  7 drops vetiver essential oil (*Vetiveria zizanioides*) for love, hex breaking, and luck

Add all essential oils to a 2 ml bottle to create a synergy. When the need arises, add 4 to 5 drops synergy to 1 teaspoon carrier oil.

Anoint dedicants undergoing initiation. Solitary practitioners can use this blend before self-dedication rituals. Anoint candles with it to invoke the energy of new beginnings and create a way for the new energies to manifest.

Warming War Massage Oil

Use before or after battles of all kinds to relax muscles and boost confidence, clarity, and strength.

  2 drops black pepper essential oil (*Piper nigrum*) for strength, clear speaking, stamina

  6 drops lavender essential oil (*Lavandula angustifolia*) for protection

1 drop lemon balm essential oil (*Melissa officinalis*), sacred to Diana, for uplifting

3 tablespoons sweet almond oil

Blend the essential oils in a glass container, then add sweet almond oil. Massage gently into sore muscles for a warming action. Helps relieve anxiety and increase stamina and mental acuity.

The Seeker

Before searching for community, covens, groves, or kindreds, make this blend.

10 drops black pepper essential oil (*Piper nigrum*) for protection

20 drops ginger essential oil (*Zingiber officinale*) for success

10 drops myrrh oil (*Commiphora myrrha*) for spirituality

25 drops sweet orange essential oil (*Citrus sinensis*) for luck

Combine all essential oils to create a synergy. Diffuse 1 drop of synergy in 100 ml water before meeting with potential community members.

Place 1 drop of synergy on the bottoms of your shoes before leaving home to ensure you make a good connection with the people you're going to meet. If you're anxious about the meeting, place a drop on a tissue and place in a pocket on your dominant side. Take a smell and a cleansing breath in through the nose, out through the mouth before walking in.

Blend 5 drops of synergy with 1 teaspoon carrier oil and anoint a candle for spells invoking community and spirituality.

Count Your Blessings

Diffuse this blend to see the light at the end of the tunnel.

  1 drop black pepper essential oil (*Piper nigrum*) to stimulate the mind

  2 drops Cape chamomile essential oil (*Eriocephalus punctulatus*) to relieve stress, nervous tension, and depression

  2 drops tangerine essential oil (*Citrus reticulata*) for joy

On those days when depression feels like a rockslide has buried you, reach up to the Goddess and She will be there for you. Blend drops in the above proportions into a glass or number 1 plastic bottle. Diffuse this synergy as needed.

  Note: If you don't have Cape chamomile, Roman chamomile (*Chamaemelum nobile*) is a good second choice. It has a meditative and peaceful essence.

Centering Oil

Diffuse this blend when grounding and centering.

  2 drops black pepper essential oil (*Piper nigrum*) for protection

  1 drop clary sage essential oil (*Salvia sclarea*) to calm

  1 drop lavender essential oil (*Lavandula angustifolia*) for peace

Blend all oils in a glass or number 1 plastic bottle. Diffuse this synergy as needed.

Protective Powder

Strew this magical salt around the perimeter of your home for protection.

  2 cups salt of your choice

  10 drops black pepper essential oil (*Piper nigrum*) for protection

2 tablespoons powdered white sage for cleansing

2 tablespoons powdered anise hyssop for protection

4 tablespoons cornmeal (an offering to the land)

Place salt in a large glass bowl. Add black pepper oil and stir. Add sage, anise hyssop, and cornmeal, and stir well. Strew the salt mixture around the perimeter of the home to protect all inhabitants. If protecting from a stalker, add mugwort so they may not find your home. Repeat annually.

Multipurpose Banishing Oil

Anoint candles for banishing magic of all kinds.

3 drops black pepper essential oil (*Piper nigrum*) for banishing

1 drop angelica essential oil (*Angelica archangelica*) for exorcism

1 drop patchouli essential oil (*Pogostemon cablin*) for banishing

1 drop rue-infused oil (*Ruta graveolen*) for banishing, exorcism

Optional: Pinch of sulfur powder for banishing

Optional: Piece of angelica root for exorcism

1 tablespoon sweet almond oil

Blend essential oils into a glass or number 1 plastic bottle. Add dry ingredients, if using. Add sweet almond oil last. Let the mixture sit for a week if angelica root is present.

Caution: Do not handle rue during pregnancy or if you are trying to conceive, as it is an abortifacient and can prevent conception.

Protection Garlic Pepper Butter

Spread this flavored butter on bread before baking for a protective meal.

  1 teaspoon black peppercorns for protection

  1 teaspoon green peppercorns for protection

  1 teaspoon white peppercorns for protection

  1 teaspoon dried garlic for protection (garlic is sacred to Hecate)

  1 tablespoon dried parsley for protection

  1 stick butter

Grind all herbs and spices in a spice mill or mortar and pestle until medium-fine. Gently fold into softened butter. If your butter is still firm from the fridge, rinse a tall glass with hot water for 15 to 30 seconds and place over the stick of butter. Leave for 30 seconds to soften. Repeat if needed. To round out the theme, try serving with a pasta dinner, as tomatoes are also protective.

Cardamom

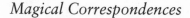

Scientific name: *Elettaria cardamomum*

Botanical family: Zingiberaceae

Origin: India

Source of plant's oil: Seeds

Evaporation: Middle note

Scent description: Warm, spicy, bright

Scent impact: Revitalize yourself and others, elevate mood

Magical Correspondences

Application: Direct inhalation

Element: Water

Day: Friday

Magical uses: Lust, fearlessness, purification, strength, focus, love, creativity

Planet: Venus

Astrological sign: Taurus

Suggested crystal: Rose quartz—ruled by Taurus and Libra: gently works to remove negativity from the chakras (energy centers in the body)

Deity/spirit: Erzulie Freda, Vodou goddess of love and women

Warnings

Do not use around children under two. It can cause breathing difficulties, spasms, or suffocation.

Herbal Lore

Known to pastry chefs as French cinnamon and "grains of paradise," this member of the ginger family has been used for centuries. The Ebers Papyrus (1550 BC), one of the oldest medical texts known to history, lists cardamom along with over 880 other medicinal herbs. Today, herbalists and aromatherapists use it to help with gas, respiratory ailments, loss of libido, acid reflux issues, erectile dysfunction, and sinus headaches.

In the realm of the magical, this spicy sister has been used in perfumes, incense, and fragrance for over three thousand years. It has been used to inflame passions and arouse lust. It has been added to wines as a potent love potion. It was ground with coffee beans in Arabic countries to warm the blood and make the heat more bearable, as it promotes sweating, and the flavor more decadent.

Uses

Place a drop of cardamom essential oil on a tissue for direct inhalation in times when focus is important. Test taking, planning, performing important tasks, and spell writing are benefitted by this oil.

Self-confidence is a trait of the successful, both in business and in romance. When approaching a love interest, making an important sales pitch, or approaching negotiations, cardamom is the best oil to choose. Diffuse 1 drop per 100 ml water while working out the wording, and carry three cardamom pods or a drop of cardamom oil on a tissue or handkerchief in the right pocket when making the presentation.

Cardamom forges mettle and encourages bravery, the ability to stand on one's own two feet. Place a drop of cardamom essential oil on the bottom of each shoe when it is time to remember to be brave and do something difficult.

To inspire creativity, add cardamom to artistic works. Venus rules not only love and lust but also beauty and the arts. See what artwork comes from a painting where a drop of cardamom is added to each paint/color used.

In a well-ventilated room, burn cardamom pods over incense charcoal or diffuse cardamom essential oil for prophecy. This works especially well for divination for love interests, or to know if a certain someone has feelings for you.

Cardamom has been used in elemental magic to evoke feelings of fire. Diffuse a drop of cardamom essential oil when meditating on meeting fire elementals. Cast sacred space starting in the south and only invite the Salamander (the elemental representing fire in the south quarter of the circle).

Mind feeling cluttered with baggage? Let cardamom do some heavy lifting. It enhances concentration and helps quiet inner static.

To enhance a partnership, bless a pair of cardamom pods and have each person carry the pod in their right pocket or on their right side for three, seven, or nine days.

Women trying to conceive can toss a handful of cardamom pods into a muslin pouch to make a bath tea. (Tip: Some stores have cheap knee-high stockings that can be turned into reusable bath teabags. Throw a few cardamom pods into the stocking and place it in the tub before filling with warm water.) Magical purification properties will help increase the likelihood of conception, and the scent can arouse male partners.

Hallowed

This blend can yield protection, focus, sanctuary, centering, and release of negative emotions.

- 1 drop cardamom essential oil (*Elettaria cardamomum*) for love, protection, focus, purification

- 2 drops neroli absolute (*Citrus aurantium*) for protection, fertility, release of negative emotions

- 2 drops sandalwood essential oil (*Santalum album*) for grounding and centering, scrying, protection, wishes, healing

Mix all essential oils in a dark-colored glass bottle. Diffuse 1 drop synergy in 100 ml water to sanctify the space before ritual.

Alternately, blend 5 drops synergy with 2½ teaspoons carrier oil and massage into skin before dedications, initiations, oaths, and vows. This combination of floral (neroli), spice (cardamom), and musk (sandalwood) is earthy and dark, and both men and women can wear this anointing oil as a perfume or cologne to protect themselves day to day.

Clarity Incense

Burn this incense to increase mental acuity, focus, and confidence.

1 teaspoon ground cardamom pods for focus

2 teaspoons dragon's blood (*Dracaena draco*) for protection, centering

½ teaspoon ground cloves for banishing hostile forces

Using a mortar and pestle, or a coffee grinder dedicated to incense preparation, grind cardamom, dragon's blood, and cloves into a fine powder. Burn over incense charcoal to increase confidence and clear thinking.

Garden of Eden

Create an oasis in the here and now.

2 drops cardamom essential oil (*Elettaria cardamomum*) for protection

3 drops lavender essential oil (*Lavandula angustifolia*) for peace, love

8 drops tangerine essential oil (*Citrus reticulata*) for peace, balance, and harmony

5 drops patchouli essential oil (*Pogostemon cablin*) for grounding, sedation

Perfect for a yoga studio, talk therapy office, or hospice, this soothing blend creates a quiet space that is loving, calm, and protected when it's diffused.

To create a calming massage oil, add 5 drops of synergy to 2 teaspoons carrier oil.

Heart Protector

Resonates with the heart chakra; purifies, protects, exorcises negative thought forms.

- 2 drops cardamom essential oil (*Elettaria cardamomum*) for purification

- 5 drops grapefruit essential oil(*Citrus paradisi*) for purification, power, generosity, heart chakra

- 1 drop rosemary essential oil (*Rosemarinus officialis*) for power, protection, purification, exorcism

- Approximately 5 drops frankincense essential oil (*Boswellia carteri*) for protection, success (see details below)

Blend cardamom, grapefruit, and rosemary. Add frankincense last, smelling the blend as each drop is added, and adjust quantity until it smells just right. This essential oil is most commonly sold as 10 percent frankincense in jojoba, so the recipe may vary depending on the brand of frankincense used.

True Faces

Use this blend to reveal treachery, discern motive, and see through glamor.

- 3 drops cardamom essential oil (*Elettaria cardamomum*) for protection, lifting spirits

- 1 drop basil essential oil (*Ocimum basilicum*) for exorcism

- 5 drops benzoin essential oil (*Styrax tonkinensis*) to reveal treachery, purify

- 1 drop cypress essential oil (*Cupressus sempervirens*) for wisdom

Diffuse 1 drop of synergy in 100 ml water before discerning the truth. Place 1 drop of synergy on a dark bowl of water for water scrying.

Add 4 drops of synergy to 2 teaspoons carrier oil to anoint candles and reveal hidden motives.

Note: Those who are prone to seizures should omit basil essential oil.

Anger into Action

Transform fury into productive outlets.

- 1 drop cardamom essential oil (*Elettaria cardamomum*) for clarity, lifting mood, protection
- 1 drop ginger essential oil (*Zingiber officinale*) for power
- 5 drops neroli essential oil (*Citrus aurantium*) to release anger, sedate, and protect
- 2 drops petitgrain essential oil (*Citrus aurantium*) to transform negative emotions, summon physical energy, and purify
- 7 drops sandalwood essential oil (*Santalum album*) for soul work, sanctifying, grounding

This is the perfect blend for when you are so angry you have to scrub the floors, or tear your hair out. Synergy can be diffused during cleaning to come back to earth. Combine all essential oils and add to 1 ounce sweet almond oil for self massage after a good "rage clean."

Citrus aurantium

Neroli, petitgrain, and bitter orange all come from *Citrus aurantium* and blend beautifully together. Neroli is solvent extracted from the flowers of the bitter orange tree. Bitter orange oil comes from the expressed rind of the fruit. And petitgrain oil originates from the distillation of the leaves and twigs of the bitter orange tree.

Bitter orange essential oil is used for relief from anxiety. Petitgrain is a fabulous wound healer. Neroli relieves stress like no other. If you have a recipe that calls for neroli but have none on hand, petitgrain can be substituted. If you have a recipe that calls for bitter orange and you are not certain whether or not it is cold pressed (phototoxic) or steam distilled (sunsafe), the same aromatic benefit can be obtained from neroli or petitgrain essential oils. (For more information, see Neroli.)

Other Realms

Diffuse for journeying, to protect and aid divination.

3 drops cardamom essential oil (*Elettaria cardamomum*) for protection, lifting mood, mental clarity

2 drops angelica essential oil (*Angelica archangelica*) for protection, uncrossing

15 drops melissa essential oil (*Melissa officinalis*) for success, lifting spirits

30 drops neroli oil (*Citrus aurantium*) for protection, sedation, release from tension

5 drops oakmoss absolute (*Evernia furfuracea*) for clairvoyance, divination

Combine all oils and diffuse 15 to 20 minutes before beginning journeying work.

Note: This recipe calls for significantly more melissa and neroli than the other oils because melissa and neroli are frequently diluted to make their price point palatable to the average consumer. If you have undiluted oils, use less. Instead of 30 drops of neroli, try 3 and see if the blend is enjoyable. Instead of 15 drops of melissa, try 1 or 2.

As hearty and plentiful as the foliage on lemon balm is, melissa essential oil is made from the flowering tops of the plant, rather than the leaves, leaving the bulk of the output usable for herbal medicine, but not essential oil. Always know the essential oil supplier. Angelica is phototoxic and should also be avoided by pregnant women and diabetics.

Cedarwood

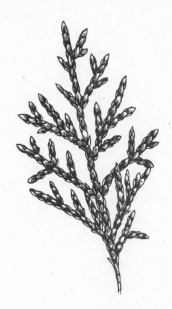

Scientific names: Atlas cedar (*Cedrus atlantica*). **Also:** red cedar (*Juniperus virginiana*); Texas cedarwood (*Juniperus mexicana*); western red cedar (*Thuja plicata*)

Botanical family: Pinaceae

Origin: Algeria, Syria, Turkey, Morocco, United States

Source of plant's oil: Bark

Evaporation: Base note

Scent description: Dry, brown, musky, smoky, spicy

Scent impact: Stimulate the emotional center of the brain, calming

Magical Correspondences

Application: Direct inhalation, diffuse, diluted topically

Elements: Fire, Air

Days: Sunday, Wednesday

Magical uses: Purification, longevity, health, protection, luck, banishing

Planets: Sun, Mercury

Astrological signs: Leo, Gemini, Virgo

Suggested crystal: Lepidolite—ruled by Libra: relieves emotional stress

Deities/spirits: Ra, ancient Egyptian sun god; Jupiter, Roman god of the sky and thunder and king of the gods

Warnings

Dilute heavily, potential sensitizer. Do not use if you are pregnant.

Herbal Lore

There are several varieties of cedar, so pay attention to labels. Cedarwood essential oil is usually distilled from the leaves, but some suppliers extract oil from cedar wood or bark. If this is the case, the bottle will be labeled as such. All cedar oils are used similarly for magical aromatherapeutic purposes.

The aromatic applications of cedarwood in emotional aromatherapy are to relieve stress, help ease depression, banish stress-induced insomnia, and promote a spiritual mind-set.

In antiquity, before books were written on paper and bound, the written word was stored in cedar trunks because the strong scent of cedar kept pests away from the precious parchment and vellum scrolls. If something was a great work of literature, it was said to be "worthy of being encased in cedar." Thus begin the tales and associations of cedar protection. Cedar protected not only the written word but anything precious. Cedar chests were discovered at the Temple of Apollo at Utica. Carbon dating on the wood revealed that the chests were over two thousand years old.

The protective qualities of cedar extend to humans as well. The skins of animals (calves, goats, and sheep), where parchments and vellum originate, have a similar composition to human skin. Cedar coffins and caskets gained popularity when the preservative nature of these funerary objects was discovered.

Uses

A dilution of 0.5 percent is suggested for potentially sensitizing oils like cedarwood, cinnamon, and clove. One drop of cedarwood essential oil in a 10 ml roller bottle filled with carrier oil will make it handy to use.

Place a drop of diluted cedarwood on your third eye for psychic protection that does not leave the subject blocked off to beneficial information.

Use diluted cedarwood essential oil as an all-purpose anointing oil; its purifying and sanctifying properties are perfect for candles, talismans, mojo bags, and divination tools.

Cleanse the air before prayer, ritual, and magical workings of all kinds and spell work (with or without circle casting) by diffusing one drop of cedarwood essential oil in 100 ml water.

Blocked energy center or chakra in the body? Try anointing that center with diluted cedarwood oil. (Remember to patch test before applying to sensitive skin.)

To banish nightmares, place a drop of cedarwood essential oil on a tissue and place inside pillowcase before bed.

To purify yourself of caustic emotions, diffuse 1 drop cedarwood essential oil in 100 ml water or anoint your heart with diluted cedarwood oil.

For emotional balance, anoint a pocket-size tigereye with diluted cedarwood essential oil and carry it in emotionally turbulent times.

To bring prosperity and luck, place a drop of cedarwood on the bottom of each shoe before leaving the house.

For increased satisfaction, carry a sprig of cedar in a cotton bag, either on a cotton cord around the neck and beneath clothing, or in a pocket. Alternately, place a drop of cedarwood essential oil on a tissue and place that inside a cotton bag. Simply anointing a tissue with oil and carrying it is not suggested, as pure essential oil is sensitizing and can cause irritation on hands entering pockets or on legs through the pocket.

The purification properties of cedar are at your fingertips; simply anoint wrists with diluted cedarwood essential oil before networking events where frequent handshakes are expected. The negative people in the room will avoid the uplifting scent of the cedar. As a bonus, it will help with pre-event jitters and nervousness.

Stretching your clairvoyant wings? Diffuse a drop of cedarwood essential oil in 100 ml of water before beginning. Gallery readings will proceed more smoothly with the smell of cedar as well.

Consecrate altars and holy spaces with diluted cedarwood. Patch test on finished surfaces first to ensure there is no discoloration.

Cedarwood wands are well suited to a variety of magic. If cedar is hard to come by, a pinewood wand anointed with diluted cedarwood oil will work. The carrier oil seals the pinewood, and the cedarwood essential oil permeates the porous pine wood.

Earthly Delights Prosperity Oil

Use this synergy to bless, petition, and harmonize finances.

2 drops cedarwood essential oil (*Cedrus atlantica*) for consecration, wealth, money, success

5 drops clary sage essential oil (*Salvia sclarea*) for prosperity, monetary retention, wealth

2 drops rose geranium essential oil (*Pelargonium graveolens*) for blessing, harmony, balance

10 drops distilled lemon essential oil (*Citrus limon*) for clarity and increased power of other ingredients

3 drops vetiver essential oil (*Vetiveria zizanioides*) for command, increased power

This earthy-smelling prosperity oil blesses all it touches. Mix all essential oils to create a synergy, and diffuse 1 drop synergy in 100 ml water or blend 1 drop synergy in 2 ml carrier oil for anointing oil.

Note: Cold-pressed lemon essential oil is phototoxic; either make sure the oil is distilled or use it out of sunlight for twelve to seventy-two hours, depending on your sensitivity.

Hex Shattering

Use to break a curse, bust a hex, and leave them in the dust.

5 drops black pepper essential oil (*Piper nigrum*) to drive away evil

1 drop cedarwood essential oil (*Cedrus atlantica*) to allow information in without harm

10 drops neroli absolute (*Citrus aurantium*) for persuasion

5 drops oakmoss absolute (*Evernia furfuracea*) for hex breaking

10 drops petitgrain essential oil (*Citrus aurantium*) for transformation

Earthy oakmoss and gentle petitgrain dance together well. Combine all essential oils for a synergy that smells amazing and unlike traditional hex-breaking blends (so no one will be the wiser).

Blend 1 drop synergy in 2 ml carrier oil for anointing oil that can be worn as perfume and a magical prophylactic to keep casual jinxes, jealousy, and the evil eye away. Or without carrier, diffuse 1 drop in 100 ml water.

Recovery

Use this blend to regain strength after an illness.

- 1 drop cedarwood essential oil (*Cedrus atlantica*) for gain, strength
- 6 drops clove essential oil (*Syzygium aromaticum*) for strength, protection
- 17 drops frankincense essential oil (*Boswellia carteri*) for purification, hex breaking
- 5 drops lavender essential oil (*Lavandula angustifolia*) for purification, sleep, longevity
- 3 drops peppermint essential oil (*Mentha piperita*) for healing, purification

Blend all essential oils. Diffuse 1 drop synergy in 100 ml water or blend 1 drop of synergy in 2 ml carrier oil to anoint candles, poppets, and mojo bags.

Psychic Defender

Use to protect the psyche and build strength in intuition.

- 5 drops cedarwood essential oil (*Cedrus atlantica*) for divination, strength
- 15 drops amber essential oil (*Pinus succinifera*) for psychic strength, success, protection

10 drops black pepper essential oil (*Piper nigrum*) to stimulate the mind, protect, drive away evil

Blend all essential oils. Diffuse 1 drop in 100 ml water during readings, meditation, or journeying. Alternately, blend 1 drop of synergy in 2 ml carrier oil for anointing oil to be used on candles, poppets, and mojo bags.

Lunar Lady

Use during lunar rituals, meditation, dedication, consecration, prayer.

7 drops cedarwood essential oil (*Cedrus atlantica*) for clairvoyance, strength

10 drops clary sage essential oil (*Salvia sclera*) for wisdom, connecting to the moon goddess, ritual work, love, calm

5 drops May Chang essential oil (*Litsea cubeba*) for meditation, prayer

Blend all essential oils. Diffuse 1 drop in 100 ml water during ritual, aspecting, divination, or prayer. Alternately, blend 1 drop of synergy in 2 ml carrier oil for anointing oil to be used on candles, poppets, and mojo bags.

Binding, Bending

Use to bind harmful people and situations.

3 drops cedarwood essential oil (*Cedrus atlantica*) for purification, strength

15 drops bergamot essential oil (*Citrus bergamia*) for commanding, success

10 drops clary sage essential oil (*Salvia sclarea*) for secrets revealed, wisdom

7 drops eucalyptus essential oil (*Eucalyptus globulus*) for binding, focus

Blend all essential oils. The topics of binding, banishing, and hexing are fraught with ethical debates, as they should be. The argument can be made that allowing child molesters, rapists, and spousal abuse to continue causes more harm than binding, banishing, or hexing the person or people involved. Food for thought. Blend 1 drop of synergy in 2 ml carrier oil for anointing candles, poppets, and mojo bags.

Hope Chest Healer

Done someone's heart wrong? Use this blend before offering them a heartfelt apology.

- 1 drop cedarwood essential oil (*Cedrus atlantica*) for purification, success
- 4 drops myrrh essential oil (*Commiphora myrrha*) for protection, good luck, success
- 4 drops petitgrain essential oil (*Citrus aurantium*) for purification, joy, transforming negative emotions
- 3 drops vanilla absolute (*Vanilla planifolia*) for love, power, passion, deep thought

When healing a bruised heart, vulnerability helps. Mix all oils into a 2 ml bottle and top with vanilla-infused oil (see Infused Oils section on pages 25–27). To be used on candles, poppets, and mojo bags. Diffuse synergy to release feelings of grief.

Chamomile

Scientific name: Roman chamomile (*Chamaemelum nobile*); German chamomile (*Matricaria chamomilla* or *M. recutita*); Cape chamomile (*Eriocephalus punctulatus*)

Botanical family: Asteraceae

Origin: United States, Egypt (Cape chamomile: South Africa)

Source of plant's oil: Flowers

Evaporation: Middle note

Scent description: Herbal, apple-like, green, sunny

Scent impact: Chamaemelum nobile: Release depression, anxiety, and insomnia; relieve stress responses in the body. *Matricaria recutita*: Achieve emotional stability, release anger, heal skin ailments. *Eriocephalus punctulatus*: Heal the heart, relieve nervous depression, relieve stress

Magical Correspondences

Application: Topical, diffuse, direct inhalation

Chamomile has two associations, and both are correct if you understand the plants:

Element: Water

Day: Monday

Magical uses: Blessing, healing, sleep

Planet: Moon

Astrological sign: Cancer

Suggested crystal: Green Calcite—ruled by Cancer: emotional balance

Deity/spirit: Hypnos, Greek god of sleep

ALTERNATE CORRESPONDENCES

Element: Fire

Day: Sunday

Magical uses: Finances, hex breaking, purification, luck

Planet: Sun

Astrological sign: Leo

Suggested crystal: Picture Jasper—ruled by Leo: inner journeys of healing

Deity/spirit: Apollo, Greek god of music, poetry, art, oracles, archery, plague, medicine, sun, light, and knowledge

Warnings

Contact a certified aromatherapist before using chamomile essential oil while pregnant. Avoid this oil if you are taking blood thinners.

HERBAL LORE

Chamomile is another plant with multiple associations depending on the source. That can be confusing for some. The color of the flowers and its bright smell lead to solar associations. Others argue that the flower is not a fiery spice or a resin, and the watery nature of the plant and its healing gifts should associate it with the moon. Both these associations have research to back them as well as multiple sources.

Since the flowers of chamomile are associated with bettering one's finances, gamblers have washed their hands in chamomile infusions to attract money. Chamomile is also added to traditional love oils to draw a mate who is generous with their finances.

In herbal medicine, chamomile is a cooling herb and is commonly recommended to subdue hot flashes, excitability, and hysteria.

Chamomile is also empowering. As such, use the aromatic oil in magic to strengthen the emotionally weak or to soothe heated tempers, anxiety, or other heightened circumstances. Other essential oils that can treat anxiety include bergamot, cedarwood, lavender, marjoram, melissa, neroli, petitgrain, rose, sandalwood, sweet orange, tangerine, vetiver, and ylang-ylang. Other empowering essential oils are bay, elemi, frankincense, myrrh, rosewood, and rosemary. The above oils can be blended with any of the chamomiles to create a scent that can nurture, empower, and soothe.

USES

Place 9 drops of chamomile oil on a cotton handkerchief and hang in the attic to protect a home from lighting strikes.

To keep away nightmares, fill a muslin tea bag with chamomile flowers or place 3 drops of chamomile on a tissue and place the bag or tissue inside your pillowcase. Drinking chamomile tea before bed can also banish nightmares.

To bring on menses, place 1 drop of chamomile essential oil in an aroma locket each day until it resumes.

To calm frazzled nerves, diffuse 1 drop of chamomile essential oil in 100 ml water.

To soothe sore muscles, blend 1 drop Roman chamomile in 1 tablespoon carrier oil and gently massage it in.

To soothe burns or alleviate premenstrual syndrome (PMS) or premenstrual dysphoric disorder (PMDD), add 1 drop German chamomile to 1 tablespoon natural aloe vera and apply to affected area. For PMS or PMDD, rub lower abdomen in gentle clockwise circles (a counterclockwise motion can discomfort bowels).

Bickering or infighting at work? Drink chamomile tea to keep those issues away from your door (or cube). Keep a sachet (preferably purple) of chamomile in your desk or near the entrance to your space. To be rewarded at work for not participating in the bickering, add a piece of hawthorn or rowan to the sachet.

To increase patience, place a drop of chamomile in an aroma locket and wear. If you don't have an aroma locket, place 3 drops on a tissue and carry it near your heart.

To prepare for magic, drink chamomile tea while grounding and centering.

For a quick purification rite, burn chamomile flowers over incense charcoal.

To bring good luck before a job interview, sales meeting, or loan proposal, wash your hands and feet in strong chamomile tea (no sugar!).

Needing physical goods? Carry a chamomile sachet in your pocket to draw the money needed to attain them.

Having a tough talk with someone? Drink chamomile tea beforehand. It will soothe anxious feelings and give you the boldness to move forward and the tenderness to carry through without cruelty.

Frayed Friend Fixer

Use this blend to soothe frayed nerves and treat depression. It's best over tea and conversation.

9 drops Roman chamomile essential oil (*Chamaemelum nobile*) or Cape chamomile essential oil (*Eriocephalus punctulatus*) for stress relief (Cape chamomile is a little pricier, but worth it!)

3 drops lemon balm essential oil (*Melissa officianalis*) for comfort (associated with Diana and the moon)

1 drop rosemary essential oil (*Rosemarinus officialis*) to soothe nerves and gain protection, love

As the caretakers of the world, we often find our kitchen table the place of confessions, tears, and long talks. Mix all essential oils in a glass bottle, and diffuse the synergy when a frantic call comes from dear friends, confused clients, or frustrated family members.

For an anointing oil that's helping during times of stress and helplessness, add 4 drops synergy to 1 tablespoon carrier oil. Your loved ones will remember time spent talking with you.

Clear Conversations

Diffuse this blend before a difficult discussion to ensure you'll be heard.

1 drop Roman chamomile essential oil (*Chamaemelum nobile*) to empower

1 drop clary sage essential oil (*Salvia sclarea*) to soothe nervousness, perform love magic

2 drops lavender essential oil (*Lavandula angustifolia*) for peace

Mix essential oils in a glass container. Use one drop of synergy per 100 ml water in diffuser.

If you don't have a diffuser, place 1 to 3 drops of this synergy on a handkerchief or tissue and breathe deeply.

Healer's Helper

Use this blend before talk therapy, massage, or reiki.

10 drops German chamomile essential oil (*Matricaria recutita*) for healing (especially skin), antianxiety

10 drops clary sage essential oil (*Salvia sclarea*) to soothe nervousness, restore balance

5 drops ylang-ylang essential oil (*Cananga odorata*) to soothe, protect health

Soft and comforting, this recipe is perfect for healing practitioners of all stripes. Blend all essential oils, and diffuse 1 drop synergy per 100 ml water.

For massage, mix 15 drops synergy per ounce of carrier oil (a good all-purpose oil is jojoba) plus a drop or two of vitamin E to preserve the mix.

Ostara Dreaming

Use this blend before bed to dream of love—especially the night before the spring equinox.

3 drops Roman chamomile essential oil (*Chamaemelum nobile*) (preferred) or Cape chamomile essential oil (*Eriocephalus punctulatus*) for luck, sleep, love

1 drop jasmine absolute (*Jasminum officinale*) for love, prophetic dreams

5 drops lavender essential oil (*Lavandula angustifolia*) for love, peace, protection

1 drop Turkish rose absolute (*Rosa damascena*) or rose geranium essential oil (*Pelargonium graveolens*) for love, dreams

Springtime is when minds drift toward love. Spring flings, first romances, and vow renewals all have their place in the spring dreaming. Mix all oils, and diffuse 1 drop synergy per 100 ml water.

For massage, mix 15 drops synergy per ounce of carrier oil (a good all-purpose oil is sweet almond) plus a drop or two of vitamin E to preserve the mix.

Let It Go!

Release that which no longer serves you with this blend.

10 drops Cape chamomile essential oil (*Eriocephalus punctulatus*) for meditation, heart healing

9 drops May Chang essential oil (*Litsea cubeba*) for meditation, rejuvenation

6 drops patchouli essential oil (*Pogostemon cablin*) for grounding, focus, love magic, sedation

The sweet, lemony scent of this blend is perfect when it is time to take a deep breath, take stock, and release those things (and sometimes people) that no longer benefit. Light and lovely in aroma, while the May Chang is soft enough to encourage meditation and relaxation.

Mix all essential oils and diffuse to release anger, increase calm, and remember what is important.

Wedding Night(ly)

Use this to keep your marriage faithful, loving, and fertile. Would make an excellent gift for newlyweds, too!

10 drops German chamomile essential oil (*Matricaria recutita*) for love, marriage

20 drops frankincense essential oil (*Boswellia carteri*) for protection, self-control

30 drops neroli essential oil (*Citrus aurantium*) for protection, fertility, antianxiety

Mix all oils into a 2 ml bottle. Diffuse 1 drop synergy per 100 ml water an hour before bed or mix 15 drops synergy per ounce of carrier oil for touch therapy.

Note: German chamomile, frankincense, and neroli are commonly diluted oils, so smell the blend as it is being made and allow for fluctuations in dilution rates between brands.

Luck Luster

All that glitters *is* gold with this blend.

5 drops German chamomile essential oil (*Matricaria recutita*) for luck

10 drops bergamot distilled essential oil (*Citrus bergamia*) for success, increased cash flow

1 drop eucalyptus essential oil (*Eucalyptus globulus*) for protection, cleansing of bad vibes

3 drops sandalwood essential oil (*Santalum album*) for wishes, protection

Mix all oils, and diffuse 1 drop of synergy in 100 ml water before going out.

Alternatively, add 3 drops synergy to 1 teaspoon vodka or rubbing alcohol and dab it on your palms.

Note: Cold-pressed bergamot is phototoxic, so do not use it before going out into direct sunlight. Use distilled or bergaptene/furanocoumarin-free whenever possible.

Cinnamon

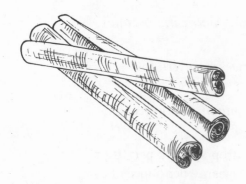

Scientific name: *Cinnamomum verum* (formerly *C. zeylanicum*)

Botanical family: Lauraceae

Origin: Indonesia, Sri Lanka, Madagascar, India

Source of plant's oil: Leaves or bark

Evaporation: Middle note

Scent description: Dark, musky, warm, spicy

Scent impact: Turn the mind to love, lust, home, and prosperity

Magical Correspondences

Application: Diffuse, direct inhalation with caution (can irritate nasal passages if inhaled directly or often)

Element: Fire

Day: Sunday

Magical uses: Abundance, health, love, lust, prosperity, attraction (physical objects, wealth, and romance)

Planet: Sun

Astrological sign: Leo

Suggested crystal: Fire opal—ruled by Pisces, Sagittarius, Leo, Libra and Cancer: allows stress to easily be channeled into beneficial change; tourmaline—ruled by Libra for inspiration

Deity/spirit: Aphrodite, Greek goddess of love, beauty, pleasure, procreation

HERBAL LORE

Cinnamon has a long history of beneficial use. Cinnamon bark was used in temple incenses from China to purify and sanctify the space.

The Bible mentions cinnamon four times: the Hebrews used it for consecrating the altar and other holy items as outlined in the Book of Exodus.

The Egyptians used cinnamon to purify the body. They believe it relieved excess bile, and it is still used to settle an upset stomach today. Cinnamon also treats nausea and vomiting.

The Egyptians would also use cinnamon in foot massages and foot bathing. The purifying properties of the plant were so highly regarded that cinnamon was among the preservation herbs used in the mummification process.

The scent of cinnamon has a calming effect, and nervine properties, and has been used to relax the mother during childbirth. (If you are pregnant or breastfeeding, consult a physician, herbalist, or certified aromatherapist before using essential oils.)

The powers of cinnamon leaf, bark, and oil are currently being studied in relation to reducing the number and size of tumors in prostate, lung, and breast cancers.

The burning heat of cinnamon essential oil has been added to natural pesticides.

USES

Diffuse a drop of cinnamon essential oil before starting creative projects to fuel your imagination.

A pinch of powdered cinnamon or a small piece of cinnamon bark in the wallet will attract money—especially if you ask Jupiter to bless it.

When moving into a new home, add three pinches of cinnamon under the doormat to protect and bring good luck into the home.

Cinnamon bark makes a delightful incense for purifying religious spaces. Keep a tin of fine cinnamon chips or coarse-ground cinnamon for purifying incense. Add a small piece of tourmaline to increase these properties.

Cinnamon is uplifting. Try baking something with cinnamon (even refrigerator biscuits) next time the blues set in.

Cinnamon benefits those in need of concentration. If you're on a deadline, try adding a pinch of cinnamon to coffee grounds before brewing. The extra perk can help get things back on track.

Astral travel is easier when you diffuse a drop of cinnamon essential oil in a well-ventilated meditation space.

To prevent attacks on good luck, smudge the outside of your home with cinnamon on incense charcoal. (Remember, cinnamon needs a well-ventilated area.) If you live in an apartment, boil two cups of water with a teaspoon of ground cinnamon on the stove.

To turn your home into a temple, add a drop of cinnamon essential oil to some of the purifying or sanctifying blends already listed in this book and diffuse.

To increase psychic ability, mix one part ground cinnamon to four parts ground lavender and burn over incense charcoal. Remember, less is more.

Cinnamon makes a potent charm for fast healing. Simply place small pieces of cinnamon bark in a mojo bag and carry it with you.

Fruitful Healing

Diffuse this blend in sick rooms to facilitate health and strength.

- 1 drop cinnamon leaf essential oil (*Cinnamomum verum*) for healing, success, strength

- 4 drops bergamot essential oil (*Citrus bergamia*) for peace, sleep, balance, success

- 1 drop lemon essential oil (*Citrus limon*) for healing, health, purification, physical energy

- 5 drops petitgrain essential oil (*Citrus aurantium*) for purification, joy, physical energy

- 2 drops vetiver essential oil (*Vetiveria zizaniodes*) for protection, grounding

Diffuse 1 drop synergy in 100 ml water in sickrooms as long as it's not contraindicated for the person's care. Check with a doctor if serious illness or other factors present themselves.

Note: Vetiver and cinnamon can be sensitizing on the skin. Use care when dispensing synergy. Wash hands throughly if synergy comes into contact with skin.

Lady Lust Massage Oil

Try out this aphrodisiac massage oil on a loving partner.

- 1 drop cinnamon leaf essential oil (*Cinnamomum verum*) for lust

- 2 drops cardamom essential oil (*Elettaria cardamomum*) for lust

- 4 drops tangerine essential oil (*Citrus reticulata*) to lift spirits

- 7 drops ylang-ylang essential oil (*Cananga odorata*) for sensuality, antianxiety

- 1 ounce carrier oil

The warming benefits of cinnamon leaf oil are apparent in this sensual blend.

Mix essential oils in a glass bottle or a nonreactive bowl. Add carrier oil and blend well. If using directly, make sure to place in a warm room, as cool or cold massage oils can cause a shock to the system. Store in a glass or number 1 plastic bottle.

Sacred Anointing Oil

This blend is inspired by Exodus 30:22–25: "Moreover, the Lord spoke to Moses, saying, 'Take also for yourself the finest of spices: of flowing myrrh five hundred shekels, and of fragrant cinnamon half as much, and of fragrant cane two hundred and fifty, and of cassia five hundred, according to the shekel of the sanctuary, and of olive oil a hin. You shall make of these a holy anointing oil, a perfume mixture, the work of a perfumer; it shall be a holy anointing oil."

   3 drops cinnamon leaf essential oil (*Cinnamomum verum*) to
      purify

   2 drops calamus essential oil (*Acorus calamus*) to sanctify

   15 drops myrrh essential oil (*Commiphora myrrha*) to sanctify

Anoint altar spaces, candles, ritual tools, and the like to purify and sanctify these sacred objects. (Caution: this oil is very hot. Use caution, and wash your hands thoroughly afterward.)

Add all essential oils in a 2 ml bottle and top with jojoba oil. When desired, add 1 to 2 drops base oil to 2 ml olive oil. Olive oil has a short shelf life, especially in warmer climates, so make small batches.

Note: This recipe is formulated using myrrh 10 percent in jojoba. With the uncut oil, much less is needed to attain the desired effect. Adjust recipe as needed.

Bless This House Floor Sweep

Sprinkle this blend over floors to bless and cleanse your home.

- 3 drops cinnamon leaf essential oil (*Cinnamomum verum*) for purification
- 2 drops frankincense essential oil (*Boswellia carteri*) for blessing
- 1 tablespoon ground catnip for love charms
- 1 tablespoon ground chicory root for uncrossing
- 1 tablespoon ground lavender for love
- 1 tablespoon ground rosemary for blessing
- 2 tablespoons ground sage for purification
- 3 cups coarse sea salt for purification

Add cinnamon and frankincense to a glass bowl. Stir well with wooden spoon. Add sea salt and stir well. Add remaining herbs, stirring thoroughly after each addition.

Wearing a dust mask, apply mix to floors. This blend should not stain rugs, but patch test first to be sure. If damage is feared, substitute whole herbs for powdered. Store mix in an airtight container when not in use.

Strong Roots

Diffuse this warm, citrusy blend to set and protect roots.

- 3 drops cinnamon leaf essential oil (*Cinnamomum verum*) for strength
- 9 drops benzoin essential oil (*Styrax tonkinensis*) for purification, revealing hidden truths
- 5 drops May Chang essential oil (*Litsea cubeba*) for strength, light heart

6 drops oakmoss absolute (*Evernia furfuracea*) for
   clairvoyance, to protect finances

1 drop rosemary essential oil (*Rosmarinus officinalis*) for
   purification, protection

Benzoin is not just another purification resin; it purifies and tears away falsehood and hidden motives. Cinnamon is the inherent strength to keep what belongs to you. May Chang elevates what could be a dark and mysterious oil. It is a reserve of strength when all hope is lost, for it is hope itself. Oakmoss lends sight to the user to see trouble coming, and protect wealth and property. Rosemary wraps all this in a neat bow with the purification and protection double whammy.

Diffuse 1 drop synergy per 100 ml water.

Clary Sage

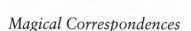

Scientific name: *Salvia sclarea*

Botanical family: Lamiaceae

Origin: France, United States

Source of plant's oil: Flowers, leaves

Evaporation: Middle note

Scent description: Soft, herbal, musty

Scent impact: Relieve stress

Magical Correspondences

Application: Diffuse, direct inhalation, and diluted on the skin

Elements: Air, Earth

Days: Monday, Wednesday

Magical uses: Dreaming, wisdom, secrets, euphoria, lunar rituals, love, ritual consecration, prosperity, retention of physical goods

Planets: Mercury, Moon

Astrological sign: Gemini

Suggested crystal: Aquamarine—ruled by Gemini: courage, protection, mental preparedness

Deity/spirit: Hypnos, Greek god of sleep

HERBAL LORE

Clary sage is a good ally in an emergency. It calms in a way that allows the subject to deal with the situation at hand in a triage protocol. The most important problem gets handled first and allows smooth flow of information without panic.

Clary sage is used largely because the common garden sage (*Salvia officinalis*) can be safely used only in small amounts. Clary sage is commonly used to help hormone levels in women. It is commonly added to aromatherapeutic blends to ease premenstrual symptoms. This does not mean that men cannot see the magical benefit of this incredible ally. The magical uses for this distinctive-smelling plant are long and illustrious.

The mental powers over dreaming, wisdom, sleep, secrets, memory, knowledge, and divination align clary sage with the element of air. The physical attributes of clary sage—its rule over prosperity, monetary wealth, material objects, and retention of worldly goods—associate it with earth.

The maternal-like energy of clary sage is the perfect base for floral perfumes and aromatic therapies.

Uses

Place a drop of clary sage essential oil on a notecard where material goods are listed to help with their manifestation. Then make sure you do the work to gain these items.

Clary sage carries the energy of knowledge. If returning to school, place a drop of clary sage essential oil on the corner of the syllabus for each class to remind you of your dedication to knowledge. The calming effect of clary sage will also help calm and prioritize tasks when it comes time for finals.

Consider the energy of prosperity in clary sage. Start a prosperity jar. Every time a smart money decision is made, make a donation to the jar. Write yourself a check, and keep it in the jar. Put spare change and small bills in there as well. Every few months or so, add a drop of clary sage essential oil to the jar. Those funds add up. Reward yourself with a vacation, a long-awaited gadget, or get even smarter and deposit it into the bank.

When life gets overwhelming, diffuse a drop of clary sage essential oil in 100 ml of water. With meditation, it will help restore the balance in your life.

Keep thieves from taking off with precious items. Where safe, anoint precious items with clary sage. Place a drop of clary sage essential oil on a tissue and place inside jewelry boxes, precious books, and the like. (Use common sense regarding anointing electronics, or anything that can be damaged by oil, like the finish on furniture.)

Wealth is not merely about prosperity; it is about the ability to feel confident in knowing where your next meal, mortgage payment, and car payment are coming from. Sit down and plan out a budget for financial independence. Diffuse clary sage during the process, and feel free to draw sigils on it, anoint it with clary sage, or make copies for intention work on vision boards. Consider a real-world budget and a goal budget for magical workings.

No matter how close we are to the people around us, tensions arise occasionally. If you live in the same house, diffuse clary sage in common areas to soothe tempers and restore balance before approaching. If you live in separate places, invite them over to talk it out. Allow tensions to cool, and when heads are clearer approach the situation. Don't wait too long, though; allowing hurt feelings to fester can destroy relationships over simple matters that commonly are not the root of the issue.

Is there a potentially harmful secret lurking? Write down the situation on a piece of paper (flash paper is best). Anoint with a drop of clary sage and burn the paper. Within twenty-four hours the truth will be known. If nothing happens after two weeks, repeat. If the secret is yours, let it out. Carrying secrets quickly wears on the soul.

To aid psychic development of clairvoyant techniques or other divination skills, consider turning to clary sage. If you keep tarot cards in a special cloth, add a dab of essential oil on the fabric to cleanse the cards and connect the user to the air of the Divine. If a crystal ball or other stone medium is used, place an anointed tissue inside the box where it is kept. Try water scrying with a drop of clary sage essential oil in a dark-colored bowl of water. The oil will sit on top of the water and release the scent as well as create a focal point to allow the mind to wander.

Memory issues? Carry a tissue with a drop of clary sage on it in your pocket. When it comes time to make a mental note, smell the tissue. When it is time to recall the information, reach for the tissue again. This practice creates a link in the scent-focused parts of the brain (the oldest part of the brain) and makes it easier to recall the information.

Knowledge is learning something every day. Wisdom is letting go of something every day.

—Zen proverb

If you are seeking clarity on a subject or making a difficult decision, go the hands-on route. Dilute a drop of clary sage essential oil in carrier oil in a 10 ml roll-on bottle and anoint your pulse points. Then grab a favorite pen and make a list of pros and cons for doing and not doing the action in question. Once a choice has been made, feel free to burn the lists to cement the choice.

Clary sage can not only help with the knowledge needed to live a fruitful life but also help with the wisdom to let go of things that do not truly matter in this life. Gently inhale clary sage essential oil wafting from the bottle. Relax your shoulders and think of one thing to let go of, even if it's only for today.

Money, Honey

Bless your financial standing with success and fortune.

18 drops clary sage essential oil (*Salvia sclarea*) for wealth

40 drops distilled bergamot essential oil (*Citrus bergamia*) for success

6 drops clove bud (*Syzygium aromaticum*) for luck (clove leaf is less intense, with a softer nose)

6 drops vetiver essential oil (*Vetiveria zizanioides*) for grounding, making the luck last

This recipe will fill the 2 ml bottle with synergy. Diffuse 1 drop synergy in 100 ml water. If using non-phototoxic oils, dilute 5 drops in 10 ml of carrier oil in a roller bottle for anointing oil that can be used on skin, or anointing candles, mojo bags, charms, talismans, and more.

Clean Cash

Break bad financial habits and manifest material objects.

6 drops clary sage essential oil (*Salvia sclarea*) for manifestation, prosperity, retention, wealth, material objects

6 drops cypress essential oil (*Cupressus sempervirens*) for purification, breaking bad habits

40 drops tangerine essential oil (*Citrus reticulata*) for luck, money, and prosperity

14 drops patchouli essential oil (*Pogostemon cablin*) for prosperity, grounding

This will fill the 2 ml bottle with synergy. Diffuse one drop in 100 ml water. For anointing oil, dilute 5 drops in 10 ml of carrier oil in a roller bottle for anointing oil that can be used on skin, or anointing candles, mojo bags, charms, talismans, and more.

Note: Cypress should also be avoided by pregnant women. *Citrus reticulata* will be labeled as tangerine or mandarin, though they are the same plant.

Clove

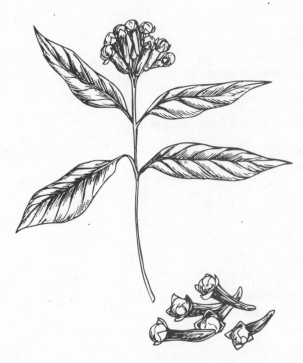

Scientific name: *Syzygium aromaticum*

Botanical family: Myrtaceae

Origin: Madagascar

Source of plant's oil: Flower buds and stems

Evaporation: Middle note

Scent description: Warm, spicy, strong, sweet, dry

Scent impact: Increase self-confidence, stimulate the mind, relax the body; encourage a sense of strength, courage, and protection

Magical Correspondences

Application: Direct inhalation, dilution

Element: Fire

Day: Thursday

Magical uses: Healing, courage, protection, fertility, purification, safe travel, blessing

Planet: Jupiter

Astrological sign: Sagittarius

Suggested crystal: Herkimer diamond—ruled by Sagittarius: tap into the energies of a person, place, or object and discern truth

Deity/spirit: Maat, ancient Egyptian goddess of truth, justice, balance, morality

The associations listed are for classical astrology. However, clove also has contemporary astrological associations presented by other noted scholars. Uranus, discovered in 1781, is one of the outermost planets, and as the outermost planets were discovered much later, those planets have fewer associations in magic and astrology. It is common to see the outermost planets sharing duty with an inner ring planet. This information above is correct for both sets, even if it seems contradictory.

The contrary information is thus:

Element: Air

Day: Wednesday

Magical uses: Memory, intellect, stopping gossip, psychic enhancement, divination

Planet: Uranus

Astrological sign: Aquarius

Suggested crystal: Kunzite—ruled by Scorpio, Taurus, and Leo: benefits loving communication

Deity/spirit: Merlin, teacher and wise man: call on him to develop intuitive senses

Warnings

Anticoagulant effects increase with warfarin, aspirin, and other drugs. Can be irritating to the skin and mucosal membranes. Even with a one-to-four ratio, test a small patch before applying to larger areas of skin. Use with caution; it can trigger contractions in pregnant women.

Herbal Lore

Clove can be used for both fiery workings and ones designed for thought and intellect. Learn all you can about both sets of information, and use clove when intuition calls for it. If you are unsure of which association to use, meditate on the working, ask a peer or teacher, or consult a pendulum or other divination method.

Clove buds have several uses medically, emotionally, and magically. A search in medical text references turned up over thirty-five papers resulting from studies on the effects of clove. It is used in many blends because of the varied use and history of the plant and oil. Many people only know clove from its reputation for soothing and numbing the pain of toothaches. The essential oil also combats aging, relieves arthritis pain, soothes lung infections, and is antiparasitic.

Historical lore suggests that cloves are so protective, they were named after nails. Stories suggest placing a small bag filled with cloves near a sleeping baby to protect it, and stringing cloves on red thread and hanging it near the baby's crib to protect them from sibling rivalry. Orange and clove pomander balls are commonly seen during the winter months to protect homes and families by warding off sickness.

Uses

Place diluted clove oil on a taper candle with the word "gossip" carved into it. Burn the candle to dispel gossip in your name and let the truth be heard. Alternately, substitute the name of the gossip in question, if known.

Use diluted clove oil to anoint doors, windows, and the backs of mirrors to protect the occupants of the home from maliciousness or astral spying.

The flower meaning of clove is dignity. Place a drop of clove essential oil on a tissue and inhale the aroma before making an apology.

Clove can help turn aside nasty weather. If damaging storms are expected, buy a small jar of whole cloves and masonry nails from the hardware store. Place the cloves at the four corners of your lawn and along the border. Then anchor the four corners with masonry nails.

Anoint the nails with diluted clove oil before sinking them into the dirt to protect your property. If you live in an apartment or condo, place cloves in the four corners of your apartment.

Strength of the Goddess Oil

Diffuse this oil to banish hopelessness and anxiety and increase courage.

  6 drops clove essential oil (*Syzygium aromaticum*) to encourage feelings of courage and protection

  6 drops black pepper essential oil (*Piper nigrum*) to ward off fatigue and empower

  9 drops frankincense essential oil (*Boswellia carterii*) to combat depression

  16 drops lavender essential oil (*Lavandula angustifolia*) to banish nervous tension

Blend all essential oils into a glass or number 1 plastic bottle, and diffuse one drop synergy per 100 ml water.

Florida Water Cologne

Create a cleansing anointing oil or spritz from this synergy.

  ¾ teaspoon clove essential oil (*Syzygium aromaticum*) for protection, exorcism

  ¾ teaspoon lavender essential oil (*Lavandula angustifolia*) for protection, purification

  ¾ teaspoon orange essential oil (*Citrus sinensis*) for purification

  1 liter 100-proof vodka or 1 liter rubbing alcohol

Pour out a tiny bit of the vodka or rubbing alcohol, and add all essential oils. Shake vigorously.

  Anoint yourself with the blend (unless you are allergic to any of the ingredients), use it as floor wash, cleanse doorways into the home, and more. Florida Water cologne has many traditional uses, and just like Mom's recipes, everyone has their own version. Some add rose, jasmine, or other Venusian herbs for a loving home to the mix as well.

Bright Business Mojo

Use this mojo to boost sales.

7 whole cloves (*Syzygium aromaticum*) to expand financial freedom

1 frankincense tear to feed the bag and keep it working

1 drop olive oil or High John the Conqueror Oil

Small red flannel bag

Optional: your business card

Bless the bag with olive oil or High John the Conqueror Oil (below) and place the cloves and frankincense inside, along with your business card, if you're using it. Charge the bag after tying or sewing it closed. Keep the mojo bag in your business's cash register (this also helps keep staff honest) or next to your skin.

High John the Conqueror Oil

2 tablespoons High John the Conqueror root, dried (*Ipomea jalapa*)

5 cloves (*Syzygium aromaticum*) for prosperity

2 cinnamon chips (*Cinnamomum verum*) for prosperity

1 small lodestone (also sold as magnetite) to draw money to you

Olive oil

Place High John the Conqueror root, cloves, cinnamon, and the lodestone into a 2-ounce bottle and top with olive oil. Remember to leave head space if you're using a glass dropper. Leave on the shelf in a dark cabinet for six to eight weeks for full effect before using. Anoint candles, cash registers, business cards, copies of contracts, and more for success in business.

Energetic Cleansing Floor Wash

Use after arguments, strife in the home, or after hosting large gatherings.

Handful of cloves to protect, cleanse

Fistful of fresh basil (*Ocimum basilicum*) or 3 tablespoons dried basil to cleanse

3 sliced lemons to brighten moods, cleanse

1 cup Florida Water Cologne to cleanse

Optional: ⅓ cup Four Thieves Vinegar (below) to protect

Place cloves and basil in a saucepan and cover with water. Bring the water to a boil and cook for 3 to 5 minutes. Remove from heat and strain water into a bucket. Add the lemons and Florida Water Cologne. Mix with a mop, using caution to avoid burning yourself. Once the water has cooled a bit, mop floors and wipe down baseboards with the blend.

Optional: set out an offering for the spirits of the land around your home.

The Four Thieves and Their Famous Vinegar

Four thieves took to robbing graves of plague victims. When they were caught by the townspeople, they were told their lives would be spared in exchange for the recipe to their vinegar. With recipes like this, everyone has their own version, some with thyme, sage, lavender, etc.

3 cloves garlic

¼ cup black peppercorns

1 teaspoon red pepper flakes

5 sprigs rosemary

1 handful fresh peppermint or ½ cup dried peppermint

1 gallon apple cider vinegar

Place all herbs into the jug of apple cider vinegar and place in a dark cabinet to age 6 to 8 weeks.

Cupid's Bow

Use this blend to purify yourself after past relationships and draw new love.

- 7 drops clove essential oil (*Syzygium aromaticum*) for protection, exorcism, love
- 6 drops clary sage essential oil (*Salvia sclera*) for love and dreams
- 10 drops lavender essential oil (*Lavandula angustifolia*) for love, protection, purification, peace

Blend oils into glass 2 ml bottle. Diffuse synergy at 1 drop per 100 ml water.

To use on candles for spell work, add 5 drops of synergy per teaspoon of carrier oil.

Yule Blessings

Good anytime of the year for protection, luck, and blessings.

- 20 drops clove essential oil (*Syzygium aromaticum*) for protection
- 20 drops of ginger essential oil (*Zingiber officinale*) for power, success
- 30 drops tangerine essential oil (*Citrus reticulate*) for luck, money

This Yule-themed oil was based on the idea of pomander balls hung around homes during the holidays to ward off cold, flu, sickness, and bad luck.

Blend all oils and diffuse 1 drop synergy in 100 ml during cold and flu season, anytime protection and luck are needed, and to bless new endeavors. To bless other projects, add 5 drops of synergy to 1 tablespoon carrier oil and anoint candles.

Drive Away Evil

Use to purge a space of evil spirits.

- 5 drops clove essential oil (*Syzygium aromaticum*) for protection, exorcism

- 5 drops basil essential oil (*Ocimum basilicum*) for exorcising, cleansing, protection

- 5 drops lemon balm essential oil (*Melissa officinalis*) for exorcism, lifting mood

- 5 drops peppermint essential oil (*Mentha piperita*) for purification, healing

Blend in 2 ml bottle and diffuse 1 drop synergy per 100 ml water in homes where spirits are not welcome. Diffuse more often in emotionally charged spaces such as therapist offices, hospice, trauma-oriented treatment centers, and clergy offices so spirits do not linger.

Coriander

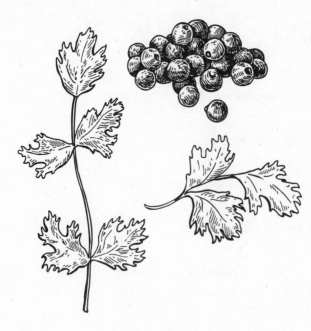

Scientific name: *Coriandrum sativum*

Botanical family: Apiaceae

Origin: India, Russia

Source of plant's oil: Seeds

Evaporation: Middle note

Scent description: Herbal, crisp, warm

Scent impact: Reassure yourself and others

Magical Correspondences

Application: Direct inhalation, diffuse

Element: Fire

Day: Sunday

Magical uses: Divination, retention, consecration, fertility, happiness, peace

Planets: Sun, Mars

Astrological sign: Leo

Suggested crystal: Petrified wood—ruled by Leo: grounding

Deity/spirit: Pele, Hawaiian goddess of fire, lightning, wind, and volcanoes

HERBAL LORE

Coriander is the seed of cilantro and a well-known addition to many styles of food, with Italian and Mexican being the most notable.

The lore of coriander frequently centers on its reputation in the realm of love, lust, and sex. Coriander seeds were frequently crushed and added to wine to act as a lustful potion, designed to inflame the loins of anyone who drank it. The seeds were not only to arouse desire in the intended target but also had a reputation for making sex last longer, and helping the coupling be healthy and fertile.

Pregnant women were told to eat coriander seeds so that they would bear intelligent children.

Wives would place coriander seeds near the hearth to release their scent, thereby increasing the peace in the home, protecting it from harm, and arousing the man of the house.

USES

Place a drop of coriander essential oil in a 10 ml roller bottle and fill with carrier oil. Anoint third eye to aid clairvoyance.

Diffuse 1 drop coriander essential oil in 100 ml of water to aid in divination.

Keep thieves from taking off with precious items by anointing them. Place a drop of coriander essential oil on a tissue and place inside jewelry boxes, precious books, and the like. (Use common sense regarding anointing electronics or anything that can be damaged by this oil.)

Use diluted coriander essential oil on a candle to reveal secrets, lies, and hidden truths.

To better communicate with animal companions, anoint your third eye and pulse points with diluted coriander essential oil and meditate on the animal in question.

To banish unwanted guests, diffuse 1 drop coriander essential oil in water or burn coriander as incense. If you use a household broom, turn the bristles up too. It will change the energy in the room, and the unwanted guests will soon leave.

Consecrate space by making this simple room spray: Add 3 drops of coriander essential oil to 1 tablespoon salt. Add the scented salt to a 2-ounce spray bottle and fill with warm water. Spray liberally to cleanse and consecrate space.

Sex magic can be a powerful use of energy. To ensure success in the bedroom, diffuse a drop of coriander essential oil a half hour to an hour before session begins.

To increase fertility, place 3 drops of coriander essential oil on a tissue and place between the mattress and box spring. If one partner is lacking fertility, anoint a pair of their underwear and place between mattress and box spring.

To increase happiness, place a drop of coriander essential oil on a tissue and carry in a pocket or close to the heart. Alternately, wear a drop of coriander essential oil in an aroma locket.

To increase the peace in a home, add 10 drops of coriander essential oil to a bucket of warm water and mop floors as normal.

To prevent illness from entering the home, add 10 drops of coriander essential oil to a bucket of warm water and wash all the doors in the home. Pour remaining water on the front porch to wash away any lingering ills.

To protect the home from all manner of ills, dilute a drop of coriander into a 10 ml roller bottle and fill with carrier oil. Anoint doors into the home as well as windows, sinks, and the backs of mirrors.

Coriander is an herb of longevity; add a drop or three to a warm bath to encourage youthful vigor.

To work with the element of fire, burn coriander herb on incense charcoal or diffuse a drop of essential oil in 100 ml water.

Working with a goddess of the moon? Coriander makes an effective base for lunar incenses as well as lunar essential oil blends.

Lunar Love

Full-moon passions run deep.

   10 drops coriander essential oil (*Coriandrum sativum*) for lust

   3 drops cedarwood essential oil (*Cedrus atlantica*) for
      purification

   20 drops neroli essential oil (*Citrus aurantium*) for sex

   1 drop rosemary essential oil (*Rosmarinus officinalis*) for lust,
      purification

Mix all essential oils and diffuse 1 drop synergy per 100 ml water.
   If out under the stars, put 3 tablespoons of water in the reservoir
of an oil burner and add 3 drops of synergy.
   This blend also makes an enticing perfume. Put 5 drops synergy in
a 10 ml roller bottle and fill to the top with carrier oil. Place on pulse
points or use as an anointing oil for candles, charms, and talismans.

Calming Communication

This blend is helpful in times of prayer, meditation, and seeking peace.

   2 drops coriander essential oil (*Coriandrum sativum*) for
      peace

   6 drops benzoin essential oil (*Styrax tonkinensis*) for balance,
      calm, harmony

   1 drop May Chang essential oil (*Litsea cubeba*) for
      meditation, prayer, mental clarity

   4 drops petitgrain essential oil (*Citrus aurantium*) for relaxing,
      purification

Mix all essential oils and diffuse 1 drop synergy per 100 ml water. To
use as perfume, add 5 drops of synergy in a 10 ml roller bottle and fill
with carrier oil. May also be used for candles, charms, and talismans.

Forgive Yourself

To truly find happiness, stop living in the past and worrying about the future.

  3 drops coriander essential oil (*Coriandrum sativum*) for peace, happiness, love, healing

  40 drops frankincense essential oil (*Boswellia carteri*) for purification, meditation, antidepressant, uplifting, spirituality

  3 drops peppermint essential oil (*Mentha piperita*) for release, renewal, uplifting

Mix all essential oils and diffuse 1 drop synergy per 100 ml water while making a list of things forgiveness is needed for. Take a break after it is complete. Take a walk, watch a sitcom, or make a cup of tea—just change the scenery for a bit. Come back to the list and the scent of frankincense and uplifting herbs. Anoint the list with a drop of synergy and burn it. Forgive yourself and pledge to change.

  To use as perfume or anointing oil, add 5 drops synergy to a 10 ml roller bottle and fill with carrier oil.

Tough Cookie

Remember your inner and outer strength with this blend.

  5 drops coriander essential oil (*Coriandrum sativum*) to prevent illness; foster inner peace, longevity

  5 drops neroli essential oil (*Citrus aurantium*) to soothe, calm, protect

  5 drops ylang-ylang essential oil (*Cananga odorata*) to calm, balance, strengthen the spirit, harmonize

Subtle floral fragrances meet with spicy coriander to remind the subject that they are so much stronger than they give themselves credit for.

Mix all essential oils and diffuse 1 drop synergy per 100 ml water to help friends in emotional crisis, or to help yourself when facing challenges and steep odds.

To use as perfume or anointing oil, add 5 drops synergy in a 10 ml roller bottle and fill with carrier oil.

Preternatural Prowess

Increases mental clarity for divination and strengthens spiritual connections.

5 drops coriander essential oil (*Coriandrum sativum*) for divination

15 drops oakmoss absolute (*Evernia furfuracea*) for divination, contacting other planes, manifestation

5 drops May Chang essential oil (*Litsea cubeba*) for journeying, mental clarity

10 drops petitgrain essential oil (*Citrus aurantium*) for transformation, relaxing, energy

This formulation is similar to the Calming Communication blend, but doubling the petitgrain makes it more uplifting while also more readily resonating with the third eye. Oakmoss adds notes of violet and leather to this otherwise bright oil. This deep absolute keeps the body grounded while the mind visits far-off realms and manifests those desires in the here and now.

Mix all essential oils and diffuse 1 drop synergy per 100 ml water. To use as perfume or anointing oil, add 5 drops of synergy in a 10 ml roller bottle and fill with carrier oil.

This blend is skin safe when diluted properly. As always, patch test before applying to sensitive areas such as around the neck and décolleté.

Scrying Secrets

Use to divine the truth in obscured situations.

5 drops coriander essential oil (*Coriandrum sativum*) for divination, secrets

20 drops grapefruit essential oil (*Citrus paradisi*) for uplifting, purifying, mental clarity, scrying

5 drops ylang-ylang essential oil (*Cananga odorata*) to soothe, protect

Mix all essential oils and diffuse one drop synergy in 100 ml water while meditating, scrying, or divining.

To scry with this oil, place 1 to 3 drops synergy in a dark-colored bowl half-filled with warm water. The warmth of the water helps release the scent of the oil. The shapes created by the oil on top of the water will help to trigger thoughts, words, images, and more within the mind's eye. The dark color of the bowl will help draw the eye into its depths, rather than merely reflecting the room. Scrying is most easily accomplished in a darkened room, with few distractions. Soft music can be helpful for tuning out distractions of the day.

Eucalyptus

Scientific name: *Eucalyptus globulous*

There are over 450 varieties of eucalyptus used in aromatherapy. Some of the most popular: Lemon-scented gum tree: *Eucalyptus citrodora*. Peppermint gum tree: *Eucalyptus dives*. Blue-leaved mallee: *Eucalyptus polybractea*. Narrow-leaved peppermint tree: *Eucalyptus radiate*. Lemon ironbark: *Eucalyptus staigeriana*.

Botanical family: Myrtaceae

Origin: Australia

Source of plant's oil: Leaves

Evaporation: Top note

Scent description: Camphoraceous, cool, herbal, minty

Scent impact: Promote wellness and purification

Magical Correspondences

Application: Diffuse

Elements: Water, Earth

Day: Monday

Magical uses: Protection, banishing, purifying, healing, health, mental and physical well-being

Planet: Moon

Astrological sign: Cancer

Suggested crystal: Moonstone—ruled by Cancer: balancing

Deity/spirit: Selene, Greek goddess of the moon

Warnings

Do not use on children under six. Use with caution on children under twelve. Relaxes muscles vital for breath, but can cause suffocation. Common allergen, sensitizing essential oil.

HERBAL LORE

Eucalyptus is known as fever tree by the aboriginal cultures of Australia. This varied member of the myrtle family has over four hundred and fifty plants in the genera Eucalyptus. Only seven to ten of these four hundred plus plants are used in aromatherapy. Each eucalyptus species performs a slightly different function, and different scents can affect their magical properties slightly.

Eucalyptus radiata is commonly used with the youngest children able to use eucalyptus because of the lower 1,8 cineole content. It helps with lymph function and can facilitate lymph drainage with proper use by a trained massage therapist. It blends well with any of the grapefruit oils and bay (*Laurel nobilis*). Both bay and eucalyptus are potentially sensitizing oils, so professional supervision is important.

Eucalyptus globulous is the most common eucalyptus species used in aromatherapy. It is commonly suggested for respiratory ailments and is added to many respiratory synergies sold by essential oil companies. If the label states it is rectified, this means the essential oil underwent a second distillation for increased eucalyptol content. *Eucalyptus globulous* is the most affordable of the eucalyptus oils. The second distillation will have a slight impact on the cost, but is worth it for increased therapeutic value.

Eucalyptus citridora, or lemon eucalyptus, is aldehyde-rich and can be severe on the senses, which makes it a good bug spray. It can be effectively blended with helichrysum essential oil *(Helichrysum italicum)* for its strong anti-inflammatory properties for summertime bumps and bruises.

Eucalyptus staigeriana is another citrus-scented member of the eucalyptus family that works well as a disinfectant. Diffuse to kill airborne bacteria in a home where colds and flus are running rampant, along with judicious hand washing.

Eucalyptus dives, also known as peppermint eucalyptus, has a high eucalyptol content and is warming. It's beneficial to the respiratory system.

Eucalyptus polybractea, or blue-leaved eucalyptus, is similar in chemical composition to *E. globulous*. It is less common on the aromatherapy shelves but is sometimes used for respiratory ailments. It will cost slightly more than *E. globulous*, but the strength of the oil makes it worth it.

USES

Place eucalyptus branches in the room of someone ill to return their health. Alternately, diffuse one drop of eucalyptus essential oil as a charm to gain health. As stated above, avoid in children under six years of age, as oils rich in 1,8 cineole can cause respiratory failure in young children.

During cold and flu season, avert illness by placing a drop of eucalyptus essential oil on a tissue and putting it inside your pillowcase.

To encourage spiritual awakening, diffuse eucalyptus essential oil in spiritual spaces, meditation rooms, yoga studios, prayer meetings, and study groups.

Eucalyptus can aid in emotional stability. Diffusing eucalyptus essential oil in emotionally charged situations can help restore balance.

Eucalyptus can be used to create balance in other areas of life. Carry a tissue with a drop of eucalyptus in your left pocket. (Note: Eucalyptus is not recommended for aroma necklaces, as it can be sensitizing to delicate skin or overwhelm the nasal passages.)

Consecrate ritual or holy spaces with eucalyptus. Dried plant material can be burned as a sanctifying incense. Pro tip: dry it yourself at home. Eucalyptus bunches are sold in flower shops and grocery stores. Do not use the eucalyptus sold in craft stores, as it is preserved in glycerin.

Pests such as mice, rats, and others cannot abide the smell of this camphoraceous herb. Spray basements or crawl spaces with this blend:

3 drops eucalyptus essential oil

3 tablespoons 100-proof vodka or rubbing alcohol

Mix in a 2-ounce spray bottle, apply lid, and shake vigorously. Remove lid and fill the rest of the way with water and spray.

Use eucalyptus oil as a charm against asthma attacks in adults.

Place a drop on a tissue and keep it in your pocket to help ease anxiety.

Eucalyptus acts as a charm against disease. Cross preserved eucalyptus branches over the threshold of your home to keep disease from entering. If you're crafty, create a swag of the branches and decorate it with symbols of protection for lasting benefit.

To gain insight during the sleeping hours, hang eucalyptus branches in your bedroom or place dried leaves inside your pillowcase. Prophetic dreams may be had.

To help fight teenage angst, spray this in common areas and in your teenager's bedroom:

3 drops eucalyptus essential oil

3 tablespoons 100-proof vodka or rubbing alcohol

Mix in a 2-ounce spray bottle, apply lid, and shake vigorously. Remove lid and fill the rest of the way with water and spray.

The cleansing properties of eucalyptus are so commonly understood, it has elevated this herb to near trope status. That is thanks to it being one of the main ingredients in a commonly used chest rub for respiratory ailments. Those cleansing properties can be used physically and spiritually as well. For the physical, add 3 drops of the eucalyptus essential oil of your choice to ½ cup salt. Stir well. Place desired amount into a running bath to cleanse your body of negativity, hexes, or the evil eye. You can also add the salt mixture to a bucket of hot water to mop with when cleansing energetically.

To add the feeling of fresh air to a stale mind, diffuse eucalyptus in a well-ventilated room and mental clarity will follow. It also reduces fatigue—great for late nights at the office when a big project is due, with none of the jitters of a caffeine overdose.

The healing properties of eucalyptus are legendary. As a healing charm, it encourages not only the healing of respiratory ailments but also general health. Carrying a piece of the bark, or a dried leaf of the herb, can act as a talisman for healing broken bones and long-term ailments.

The strong, cool scent of eucalyptus can be used to awaken the inner healer as well. Reiki practitioners, yoga teachers, therapeutic touch practitioners, and shamanic practitioners can use it to recall the power of community healing and work at large. Gently sniff directly from the bottle when compassion fatigue sets in.

This plant can be used to connect to water elementals. Cast a circle and invite only water to meet a water elemental. Diffuse the eucalyptus essential oil of choice to create an elemental connection.

The scent of eucalyptus does not just increase psychic dreams; it also helps to avert nightmares. Add a handful of eucalyptus leaves to a muslin tea bag and place inside the pillow. Also encourages restful sleep.

New Bee

We were all new once. This oil is designed to calm the newly awakened.

- 1 drop eucalyptus essential oil (*Eucalyptus globulous*) for awakening, emotional balance, energy

- 1 drop lavender essential oil (*Lavandula angustifolia*) for balance, centering, harmony, protection

- 7 drops sandalwood essential oil (*Santalum album*) for balance, spirituality, psychic development, harmony

When finding a new practice, whether it's yoga, magic, or the perfect diet, people have a tendency to jump in with both feet. This can lead to temporary obsessions, talking the ear off anyone who stands too close, and annoying loved ones. This nurturing and clean-smelling synergy is well suited to diffusing around the house, as well as being used as an anointing oil on skin and on candles and charms. It helps the newbie remember to breathe, remain calm, and understand that no matter how life-changing a new practice can be, it will never be suited to every person. Take a deep breath and step back.

Mix all essential oils. Add 5 drops of synergy to a 10 ml bottle, then fill with carrier oil. Shake well and apply.

Muse Minder

This blend works well for all creative pursuits, including vanquishing writer's block.

> 5 drops eucalyptus essential oil (*Eucalyptus globulous*) for awakening
>
> 1 drop cinnamon leaf essential oil (*Cinnamomum verum*) for creativity, uplifting
>
> 3 drops oakmoss absolute (*Evernia furfuraceae*) for manifestation
>
> 10 drops tangerine essential oil (*Citrus reticulata*) for inspiration

This fusion of high eucalyptus notes and dark oakmoss grounds the mind and the heart. The tangerine and cinnamon lift the burdens of the creative mind to allow the art to flow.

Mix all essential oils and use 1 drop synergy per 100 ml water in a diffuser near creative spaces and workshops to allow art to manifest.

Use diluted oil to anoint candles. Add 5 drops of synergy in a 10 ml bottle, then fill with carrier oil. Shake well and apply.

Note: do not use this oil on skin if you are sensitive to cinnamon.

Frankincense

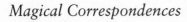

Scientific name: *Boswellia carteri*

Botanical family: Burseraceae

Origin: Somalia

Source of plant's oil: Resin

Evaporation: Base note

Scent description: Warm, earthy, slightly musky, notes of citrus on the back end

Scent impact: Engage spiritual affiliations, ease depression

Magical Correspondences

Application: Direct inhalation, diffusing, topical applications

Element: Fire

Day: Sunday

Magical uses: Purification, empower spells, justice, meditation, banishing, spirituality, consecration, strength, protection

Planet: Sun

Astrological sign: Leo

Suggested crystal: Quartz (the most prevalent mineral on the planet)—all astrological signs: ubiquity (just as quartz is everywhere, for all things, so is frankincense)

Deity/spirit: Februus, Roman god of purification

Herbal Lore

Frankincense has been used in religious, medicinal, and social applications for more than five thousand years. Frankincense is so often seen with its resin counterpart, myrrh (*Commiphora myrrha*), that people often mistake them for one resin, frankincense-and-myrrh.

Once the *Boswellia carteri* tree reaches twenty years, it is tapped in a way similar to how maple trees are tapped for syrup. Milky white tree sap begins to drip from the spigot, and when dried, the drops of resin that form are called tears. To create the signature frankincense oil that has crowned kings and queens, the resin is steam distilled to produce a dark, viscous oil. If the oil you are buying looks and feels like water, consider quality testing.

Pure frankincense is very expensive and therefore is one of the most adulterated oils on the market today. If the oil being purchased is clear and thin, it is highly adulterated. Ethical companies will state plainly on the label the dilution (e.g., "10 percent frankincense in jojoba"). See the section on quality testing essential oils for further information.

Due to the popularity of frankincense in religious and spiritual rituals, frankincense is becoming harder to obtain and is in danger of becoming endangered. Though studies have been released on the danger to this beautifully scented tree, even if entire farms were devoted to growing frankincense they would not start producing frankincense tears for twenty years. This leaves an obvious gap in the production schedule.

Medical research into the nature of frankincense has yielded information on its antidepressant qualities, especially its use in treating children with depression, as most antidepressants have the opposite effect on children eighteen and under. Frankincense is also being screened in cancer studies as an antitumor drug.

Social uses of frankincense go back over five thousand years. Ground frankincense tears were worn as eyeliner. Chewing the tears was prescribed in ancient times to treat halitosis and a number of other ailments. It was given at the birth of kings because it was said to have the ability to treat any ailment known to mankind. The healing properties of this herb were so well trusted that the Ebers Papyrus

(1550 BC) mentions it by name among the 1,877 healing prescriptions and recipes it details. A gift of frankincense was also a display of wealth, because at the time it was more valuable than gold.

The magical uses of frankincense are as many as its religious and medicinal uses combined. It crosses religious barriers to invoke feelings of sanctity, comfort, safety, and security in churchgoers and ritualists the world over.

Frankincense is more effective than white sage for banishing and purifying people, places, and things. Frankincense does not cause the divisiveness that white sage does when used by non-native peoples. (White sage is wild crafted, meaning it is harvested in the wild because it is difficult to farm, and it has become trendy in native plant medicine. This is not only insulting to native peoples but also makes it hard to find, and drives up the price.)

Frankincense has antidepressant effects: it increases emotional strength and elevates mood while still being meditative.

The alternative to *Boswellia carteri* tears and oils is *Boswellia sacra*, or sacred frankincense. Do not be concerned—all frankincense is sacred. It is merely a different cultivar of tree. The magical uses for these are the same.

USES

If you feel as though something bad has happened in your home or office, diffuse a drop of frankincense essential oil in 100 ml water, and place 4 frankincense tears in the room (one in each corner) to clear it of evil presence.

Burn frankincense tears or diffuse frankincense essential oil to connect with angelic beings.

To increase the efficacy of meditation, burn frankincense resin during your practice. (Start with a single small tear on incense charcoal. Resin smoke is notoriously thick, and it is easy to add more resin if needed.)

Planning a trip? Place a frankincense tear in a pocket for a safe journey, or anoint the bottoms of your shoes with frankincense essential oil.

Encountering a mental block to a practice? Whether it's affecting your yoga practice, magic, meditation, even going to the gym, frankincense can help. Burn the resin if desired, or diffuse the essential oil in a home or studio environment. In a gym or public space, anoint your body with 2.5 percent diluted frankincense oil. One drop in 2 teaspoons of carrier oil is the perfect amount for commercially sold 10 percent dilution frankincense essential oil.

Frankincense and its partner in crime are used in consecration rituals from religions the world over. Place 1 drop of frankincense and 1 drop of myrrh (*Commiphora myrrha*) in 4 teaspoons carrier oil and use the blend to anoint ritual tools, sacred spaces, and more. Or diffuse 1 drop of each in a room diffuser for yoga studios, religious spaces, meetinghouses, and study groups.

Frankincense represents the element of fire. Burn frankincense tears to symbolize the element of fire in spaces where candles may not be practical.

If you're looking for an oil or incense for a baby blessing, baptism, mother-to-be blessing, or wiccaning, frankincense is the one.

Frankincense can also benefit psychic development. For astral travel, burn frankincense incense. Frankincense increases spiritual abilities and psychic awareness (think of it as developing an early warning system).

Incoming!

In those moments when something doesn't feel right, don't wait for the bad thing to happen—fight back.

3 drops frankincense essential oil (*Boswellia carteri*) for purification, protection, strength, psychic awareness

3 drops lavender essential oil (*Lavandula angustifolia*) for strength, protection, purification

6 drops neroli essential oil (*Citrus aurantium*) for psychic shielding, protection, stress relief

All too often, we hear something or feel something that makes us feel as though "something wicked this way comes." Instead of waiting around to see what it is, like those people we holler at in horror movies, do something about it. Throw salt over your shoulder or light a candle. Or perhaps diffuse this union of well-intentioned oils and beat the bad before it lands.

Mix all essential oils and anoint a candle with a drop of the synergy.

None Shall Pass

Nothing is getting through this shield of allies.

- 4 drops frankincense essential oil (*Boswellia carteri*) for hex breaking
- 2 drops bergamot essential oil (*Citrus bergamia*) for commanding strength
- 3 drops lemon balm essential oil (*Melissa officinalis*) for success, happiness
- 2 drops oakmoss absolute (*Evernia furfuracea*) for hex breaking, grounding

Whereas the Incoming! blend offers protection from potential psychic attack, None Shall Pass is a preventive for bane work or hexing magic. The best way to keep from being the target of baneful magic is not to be a jerk. Barring that, people who attempt to change the world for the better collect grumpy people who want the world to stay the way it is.

Mix all oils, and diffuse 1 drop synergy in 100 ml water to shield a home, sacred space, or office. To translate this delectable-smelling oil into a perfume that can be used to keep away jinxes, curses, and the evil eye, place 5 drops of synergy in a 10 ml bottle and fill the rest of the way with carrier oil. Anoint candles, mojo bags, and charms with diluted blend for increased magical success.

Geranium (Rose)

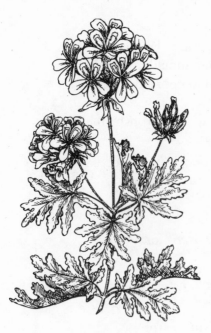

Scientific name: *Pelargonium graveolens*

Botanical family: Geraniaceae

Origin: Egypt, India, Morocco

Source of plant's oil: Leaves

Evaporation: Middle note

Scent description: Fresh, clean, herbal, sweet, floral

Scent impact: Calm intense emotions, regain balance

Magical Correspondences

Application: Direct inhalation, diffuser, dilution on skin

Element: Water

Day: Friday

Magical uses: Balance, healing, protection, love

Planet: Venus

Astrological sign: Taurus

Suggested crystal: Selenite—ruled by Taurus: awareness of mind and body, and emotional well-being

Deity/spirit: Concordia, Roman goddess of harmony

Warnings

Potentially toxic if ingested. Never use essential oils internally without the supervision of a trained professional. Commonly adulterated, use a reputable dealer to find this oil.

Herbal Lore

Seventeen species of the Pelargonium family are commonly used to create this essential oil, and *P. graveolens* is the one most often used. The medicinally used geranium species is not a Pelargonium at all. It is a true geranium, *Geranium maculatum*, or cranesbill. It is important not to confuse the two. The Pelargoniums that are used in aromatherapy have a different magical use from their medicinal counterpart, and further research is recommended.

Pelargonium graveolens is also called rose geranium because it smells similar to traditional English roses and this common garden annual. Of the seventeen species that are used to create scent, there are many wildly different versions, from spicy fragrances reminiscent of mint, nutmeg, or clove to citrusy and light ones. Because all of these scents can be derived from geraniums, they blend well with each other.

The energy of geranium, especially rose geranium, reminds us that we are whole, strong, and protected. The magic of the geraniums is not offense; it is defense. The scent of rose is uplifting and strengthening. The oil reminds us that depression, illness, and hexes are opportunistic parasites. They strike when we are at our weakest and cannot adequately protect ourselves. With this in mind, developing a working relationship with geranium should be a priority.

Think of rose geranium like echinacea. It has become common knowledge that echinacea and illness are related. However, common understanding of this powerful health ally is reversed: echinacea is not used to *cure* illness; it is supposed to *prevent* illness by boosting the immune system before sickness can occur. (See *Healing Wise* by Susun Weed for more information on medicinal herbs.)

Uses

Harmony is the hallmark of geranium. Plant a border of geranium plants around the home to stabilize those living within. Alternate with another member of the geranium family, *Pelargonium citrosum*, for a pleasant citrus and rose blend.

Diffuse a drop of geranium essential oil in water to calm tense situations. Whether it's having a tough discussion with a partner or mediating a dispute between coven members, peers, or children, it will calm the emotions of those present and help the conversation move forward. Diffuse geranium to help end arguments between people present.

Geranium can facilitate inner growth as well. Diffuse a drop of geranium essential oil in water during religious counseling sessions to help release old thought patterns.

Geranium has a reputation for healing work, both physically and emotionally. It inspires compassion as well, so it is a good long-term care essential oil, as it not only supports the healing work of the patient but also helps to stave off compassion fatigue for the caregiver.

Geranium is emotionally uplifting. Diffuse its essential oil regularly when seasonal affective disorder (SAD) is likely to creep in.

Geranium is a hearty ally for those battling emotional disturbances. It inspires courage and confidence, and a calm emotional state. It is balancing and therefore helps to alleviate depression. It can act as a temporary mood stabilizer while professional mental health advocates are arranged. Remember, magic is no substitute for professional medical services.

If things start to feel routine or stagnant at home, geranium can renew those feelings of joy. Diffuse geranium with bergamot for an uplifting treat. Just one drop of geranium and one drop of *Citrus bergamia* each will have occupants feeling a spring in their step in no time.

Geranium's scent and Venusian associations have been used in place of rose from time immemorial. Thus, it is used for love spells, fertility rites, and relationship healing.

Geranium is an easy ally to work with for hex breaking. It stimulates awareness internally and externally. It also inspires focused action in response to threats. The hex-breaking properties of geranium also make it a powerful ally for protection work. Simply place 1 drop of geranium essential oil in 2 ml of carrier oil and shake. Apply to doors, windows, and the backs of mirrors.

Geranium is not only helpful when it comes to hex breaking, it can avert the hex before it can even be cast. If you suspect someone may set a curse or hex in motion, be proactive and diffuse geranium oil in the home (and office).

Geraniums have been used in magic dealing with the fae. Diffuse the essential oil in ritual spaces where meditations dealing with the hidden folk are performed. Consider having potted geraniums in the space as well.

Devotion is another badge of geranium oil. It can be used to anoint deity statues, sacred space, and devotional candles.

Want to bring on change in a hurry? Add geranium to the spell! Growing geranium at home means a steady supply of leaves that can be dried and added to workings. Use geranium anointing oil to dress charms, mojo bags, and candles for magical fuel. Simply place one drop of geranium in 2 ml of carrier oil and shake.

Geranium can be used to banish nightmares. Diffuse it with another nightmare-banishing oil, like lavender, thirty minutes before bed to relax the mind before sleep.

Freedom Spell

The associations of Venus and hex breaking make this essential oil the perfect ally for work involving freedom. In order to grant a romantic partner freedom and healing after a breakup, anoint two candles with diluted geranium oil (1 drop of geranium essential oil in 2 ml of carrier oil). These candles can be identical tapers or different colors to represent each partner. Place the candles in candleholders and light them. As the candles burn, move them further and further apart. By the time they have finished burning, they should be in separate rooms if possible.

Letting Go Spell

Healing relationships is never easy, especially between people who are supposed to love one another. If the relationship has reached the point of no return, write the other person a letter. Pour out all those feelings. Whether it's one page or fifty pages, do not censor yourself. Get out every hurtful thing that has been carried around. Then take the letter outside, sprinkle it with a few drops of geranium essential oil, and burn it in a fire-safe container outside. Backyard fire pits, grills, and cauldrons all make a safe fire receptacle. Make sure to obey burning ordinances, especially for those in drought-ridden areas.

Daily Devotional

Use this devotional oil daily for spiritual connections.

> 10 drops rose geranium essential oil (*Pelargonium graveolens*) for spirituality
>
> 20 drops lemon essential oil (*Citrus limon*) for calming, clarity, love
>
> 15 drops sandalwood essential oil (*Santalum album*) for spirituality

Blend all essential oils in a 2 ml bottle and diffuse 1 drop synergy per 100 ml water during devotional work. Whether you are engaging in prayer, meditation, or spellwork, this oil can calm, center, and help you feel the loving support of deities in a practical setting.

Lady Liberty

Use this blend in spells for freedom, and to protect against ill health, hexes, and people.

  2 drops rose geranium essential oil (*Pelargonium graveolens*) for healing, freedom, and mood

  5 drops tangerine essential oil (*Citrus reticulate*) for inspiration, defense

  10 drops ylang-ylang essential oil (*Cananga odorata*) for calm, harmony

Blend essential oils in a 2 ml bottle and diffuse 1 drop synergy per 100 ml water to dissolve threads of entanglement. Add 1 drop synergy to 2 ml carrier oil for anointing oil for candles, charms, mojo bags, and more, for freedom, independence, inner strength, and the determination to be in control.

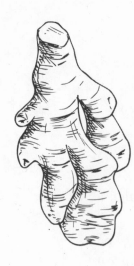

Ginger

Scientific name: *Zingiber officinale*

Botanical family: Zingiberaceae

Origin: China

Source of plant's oil: Roots

Evaporation: Base note

Scent description: Fresh, biting, and spicy

Scent impact: Empower yourself and others, gain energy

Magical Correspondences

Application: Direct inhalation, diffusion

Element: Fire

Day: Tuesday

Magical uses: Healing, beauty, courage, energy, strength, magical fuel

Planet: Mars

Astrological sign: Aries

Suggested crystal: Labradorite—ruled by Leo: healing and balancing of energies

Deity/spirit: Amaethon, Welsh god of agriculture

Warnings

Use caution when on anticoagulant drugs like aspirin and warfarin. Possible skin sensitizer.

Uses

Place a drop or two of ginger essential oil on a cotton ball inside a small jar (the size of a baby food jar or small honey jar). Keep it in your office or near your desk to energize your mind during that afternoon post-lunch slump.

For an effective healing charm, place a slice of fresh ginger in a muslin bag and empower it for healing before giving to sick friends or family.

Ginger has long been found to invoke feelings of love, lust, and sexuality. If it's time for a new, loving relationship, get some fresh ginger. Write your full name and birthday on a small piece of paper and place it between two slices of fresh ginger. Bind with red thread or ribbon and carry it in your purse. If you have access to a red or pink bag, that's ideal; if not, muslin will do.

To arouse passion, diffuse a drop of ginger essential oil in the space where the most time will be spent. Start the diffuser up to thirty minutes before arrival or expected activity for maximum effect.

Ginger makes a powerful ally. It is in the family of plants that act as magical rocket fuel for spell work. The fiery smell and action of ginger lend themselves well to spell work because of the effect on human musculature. Add dried or fresh ginger to mojo bags, charms, and spells for amplified effect. Ginger essential oil can also be of help.

Ginger helps regulate muscle contractions and is used to soothe irritations in the muscle fibers. For this reason herbalists and doctors alike have prescribed ginger capsules for menstrual difficulties. (Consult a doctor, herbalist, or aromatherapist before using anything for reported health benefits, as every human is different and has a varied medical history.)

Ginger's stimulating nature is also a boon for prosperity magic. Whether you're looking to receive repayment of a loan or improve the general financial well-being of your household, ginger can stimulate your economy in a hurry.

Since ginger is a thick, strong root with a particularly strong smell, it should not come as a surprise that this essential oil is well suited for spells involving magical and physical strength and courage. This emphatic herbal ally works well in courage spells when paired with thyme. Ginger and thyme are especially well suited to healing work involving potentially life-threatening illnesses because of the physical strength and healing embodied by ginger, and the quiet strength of thyme. Place these two dried in a mojo bag for those in need of support during a health crisis.

Are you a creative professional? Are you a graphic designer, a painter, a writer, or a jewelry designer? Let the scent of ginger help inspire the creativity inside. Diffuse a drop of ginger in creative spaces, workshops, and offices to arouse the muse within.

The prosperity magic involved with ginger can be accessed in more than one way. Add a small piece of dried ginger root to your coin purse for stimulating personal finances. Powdered ginger root can be sprinkled in a billfold as well to keep the money flowing.

Let ginger's fiery scent enliven the protection measures within the home. Place dried ginger root around the four corners of the home. Macerate ginger root in rubbing alcohol, corn liquor, or vodka for 6 weeks, and sprinkle the liquid around the perimeter of the home to ward and protect that space. Dried ginger root can be burned outside the home over incense charcoal. (Avoid burning ginger root indoors, as it can cause respiratory irritation.) If you live in an apartment or condo, boil fresh or dried ginger on the stove to release the fragrance.

The same methods for protecting your home will also purify the space of any lingering negative energies. Diffuse 1 drop ginger essential oil in 100 ml water in a well-ventilated space to clear out malicious feelings.

If you are experimenting with astral travel, try formulating a signature blend of essential oils featuring ginger. Using a signature fragrance for astral travel that is not used for other things can help create a scent trigger that helps get the mind into that space faster each time it is used.

Spells for beauty, based on the fiery lust of ginger, should be undertaken on a Friday for the best efficacy. Add a tissue with a drop of ginger essential oil on it to a cosmetics bag to imbue the cosmetics with the energy of beauty. Write a poem to a goddess of love and beauty on a nice paper or parchment and anoint with ginger oil. Each person has beauty; perhaps anoint a candle and ask a favored goddess of love and beauty to help see the inner beauty present.

Hexes don't stand a chance against fiery ginger root. Uncrossing rituals are beneficial if a direct attack is suspected from an unknown source. Anoint a candle with your name and ginger oil to break any hexes that could have been cast. Remember, true hexes are rarer than folks think; they take energy, time, dedication, and knowledge. More commonly, small jinxes and the jealousy of the evil eye are at work—those things are easily dispatched. The jealousy of a new job, a new car, and even a new love can open the door to petty people, so be on the lookout.

Self-improvement isn't only for New Year's resolutions; it should be a lifelong endeavor. Create an actionable list of ways to better yourself and anoint it with ginger oil. If the list is meant to be burned, write it on flash paper instead of regular paper, as it will go up instantly and leave no ash, smoke, or soot behind.

The energizing effect of ginger can be applied to the self or even household luck. Support the spark of luck that ginger gives with the energy of success from bergamot (*Citrus bergamia*) to give a boost. Diffuse 1 drop of ginger with 1 drop of bergamot in 100 ml water to turn the mind toward success of a monetary variety.

Strengthen Romantic Relationships

If the energizing, healing, and love aspects of ginger are considered as a whole, it should come as no surprise that ginger can help strengthen and energize romantic relationships.

Add 1 drop of ginger essential oil to 2 ml carrier oil. Shake well to blend.

To restore a lost spark, anoint a figural candle for each romantic partner. (Traditionally shaped candles work, though figural candles add more focus to the work.) As ginger has a reputation for restoring a man's lost, *ahem*, vitality, anointing the genitalia of the candle should restore him. Using a red thread, tie the figures together, facing one another, in a loving embrace. Burn candles on the full moon if possible or on a Friday night when the moon is waxing. Use extra caution as the burning thread will present increased fire hazard. Consider burning in a cauldron or high-sided pot.

To See through Emotions

Ginger is useful for discerning when our emotions have been calling the shots and pulling the wool over our eyes.

Diffuse a drop of ginger in a space where distractions and interruptions are unlikely. Sitting comfortably, close your eyes and breathe deeply. Breathe in through the nose and out through the mouth. Imagine a colored hallway with bands of red, orange, yellow, green, blue, indigo, and violet (the colors of the rainbow are useful in meditation to achieve a deeper state of consciousness). Try to see the current situation from above. Are there negative cords tying the hands of those involved? Does the space between those involved look dark, murky, or muddy? Look closer. The picture can be viewed as closely as you need. If even the thought of the meditation leads to discomfort, it is possible the answer is already apparent. If it will be helpful, record the instructions to play during the meditation. Consider playing a drumming track while recording the instructions.

Rearview Mirror

This is an empowering blend for letting go of the past and moving forward.

- 1 drop ginger essential oil (*Zingiber officinale*) for healing, courage, purification
- 8 drops bergamot essential oil (*Citrus bergamia*) for commanding strength, success
- 2 drops petitgrain essential oil (*Citrus aurantium*) for transformation, purification, banishing depression
- 1 drop rosemary essential oil (*Rosemarinus officinalis*) to release negative emotions, transform, meditate, elevate mood

Magic is an important practice because it bestows agency. It allows us to refuse to accept the cards we have been dealt. Magic gives us tools to create change in our lives. Magic is empowering. That being said, magic is no replacement for qualified therapeutic intervention. They go hand in hand.

Mix all essential oils and diffuse 1 drop synergy per 100 ml water. For an anointing oil, mix 1 drop with 2 ml carrier oil.

To practice overcoming an obstacle or problem, try this version of poppet magic, a crafting project that uses Rearview Mirror anointing oil: First, draw a gingerbread man on doubled-over fabric or paper. Cut out the gingerbread man. Using permanent marker, draw or write what needs to be put in the rearview. Sew or staple the two pieces together, leaving a 1- to 2-inch hole. Stuff the gingerbread man, and then close the hole. Anoint the figure with Rearview Mirror anointing oil. Once the gingerbread is recognizable as the problem, destroy it: tear it up, cut it up with scissors, or if it is paper, burn it. If the materials are all-natural and biodegradable, throw them into a swiftly moving body of water. Dispose of any parts or remnants off the property, and say, "I put it behind me." Stomp your dominant foot three times and walk away without looking back. If talk therapy has not begun, consider it now.

Further reading: *The Body Keeps the Score: Brain, Mind, and Body in the Healing of Trauma* by Bessel van der Kolk, MD.

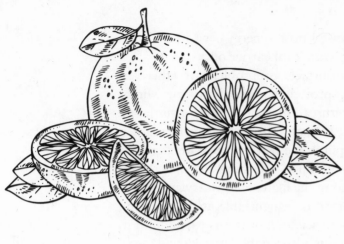

Grapefruit

Scientific name: *Citrus paradisi*

Botanical family: Rutaceae

Origin: United States

Source of plant's oil: Peels

Evaporation: Top note

Scent description: Bright, sweet, citrusy

Scent impact: Elevate mood

Magical Correspondences

Application: Direct inhalation, diffuser, topical (use with caution)

Element: Air

Day: Sunday

Magical uses: Healing, cleansing, protection, uplifting, purification

Planet: Sun

Astrological sign: Leo

Suggested crystal: Citrine—ruled by Gemini, Aries, Libra, and Leo: directs personal power and creativity

Deity/spirit: Alectrona, Greek goddess of the sun and the morning

Warnings

Cold-pressed grapefruit oils are phototoxic. If blends will be worn in the sun, wait twelve to seventy-two hours after application to go outside, depending on sensitivity. Distilled grapefruit is not known to be phototoxic and should be patch tested for sensitivity before using in the sun. It will have a different color and a slightly different aroma from the cold-pressed essential oil, but is much safer for topical use. If the blend is to be diffused only, use cold-pressed grapefruit essential oil.

Herbal Lore

As grapefruit is a modern hybrid of sweet orange (*Citrus sinensis*) and pomelo (*Citrus maxima*), there is little lore and history for its use. Instead of discounting the magical contributions of grapefruit in its relatively short time on earth, let's look at the histories of the pomelo and the sweet orange to create a new magical dynasty with a destiny of its own. The magical uses of grapefruit essential oil are of both fruits.

Uses

Place dried grapefruit rind scented with a few drops of grapefruit essential oil on the bedside table of a sickroom to lend healing energies to the ill person.

Grapefruit is an interesting ally for protection. Instead of merely forming a protective egg or sphere around the protected, grapefruit's solar energy burns away the threads of the threat to friends and loved ones. Simply add a drop of grapefruit oil to cotton and place it in an aroma locket before sending a loved one out into the world. Adding another protective essential oil such as lavender or frankincense will make the effect even stronger.

The bright scent of grapefruit is ideal for encouraging the development of self-esteem. It raises the vibration of the person as a whole and strengthens the self until the user no longer needs the support and can stand on their own two feet. Wear or carry a scented tissue in a pocket on days when the effort seems like more than the reward.

The uplifting reputation of grapefruit is well deserved. The sweet aroma is due to the sweet orange half of its parentage. Citrus oils have a long history of strength, power, and prestige in the world of aroma. Tangerine/mandarin essential oil is one of the few listed for magical defense—with this little power plant, not many others are needed. Diffuse a drop of grapefruit during your morning wakeup ritual—you'll find that even Mondays turn out brighter.

The hormone-regulating magic of grapefruit is well known. It not only dissipates hormone-related irritability, it can even soothe the symptoms of menopause. Consider a gently scented grapefruit spritz for magically banishing premenstrual symptoms and menopause difficulties.

Grapefruit is an essential oil that banishes depression and lifts the spirit. It inspires the clarity and knowledge that everything will be all right even if it doesn't feel that way at this moment. Diffuse grapefruit essential oil when joyful events are happening, so that when a boost is needed the scent can inspire that same level of joy without effort.

Grapefruit is the scent of renewal. Charm bags filled with grapefruit peel scented with grapefruit essential oil are a lovely gift for (sabbat) celebrations involving renewal and rebirth. The first day of spring is the perfect time to get in touch with the energy of renewal.

Acidic citrus juice is being studied for use in batteries, and this energy can easily apply to your magical practice. Anoint candles with diluted grapefruit essential oil (1 drop per 2 ml carrier oil) to provide a magical boost to workings. Anoint charms, mojo bags, talismans, and more to gain a boost of energy. Even the scent of the oil will provide a quick pick-me-up. Just remember, no essential oil is a replacement for a good night's rest.

If sincere and direct focus is needed, grab the bottle of grapefruit essential oil for an easy boost. It's great for study sessions, directed learning, or guided meditations. Diffuse 1 drop per 100 ml water during the session.

Purification is the seal of all citrus fruits. For a quick and easy ritual purification bath, grab 2 tablespoons of a favorite salt and add 5 drops of grapefruit essential oil. Stir thoroughly with a nonreactive implement, such as a wooden spoon. Sprinkle the mixture into a running warm bath and enjoy the purification before the big event.

All of this uplifting talk of grapefruit can also apply to energy within the body, sometimes referred to as *chi* or *qi*. Raising the vibrations within the body can make it easier to engage in spiritual work such as prayer, intuitive readings, meditation, and praise. Direct inhalation of grapefruit essential oil from a tissue or diffusion in the working space is a quick and easy way to bring up the energy in a room.

A quick waft from the grapefruit oil bottle can also ease tension that causes headaches, as it's related to psychic power, strength, and intuition.

Chill Out, Cheer Up!

Use this blend to allow cooler heads to prevail.

3 drops grapefruit essential oil (*Citrus paradisi*) to heal, protect, renew

3 drops lavender essential oil (*Lavandula angustifolia*) for harmony, peace, strength

3 drops peppermint essential oil (*Mentha piperita*) to purify, release, lift

2 tablespoons witch hazel

Place essential oils and witch hazel in a 2-ounce pump spray bottle. Cap it and give it a good shake. Unscrew the cap and fill the rest of the way with cool water. Spritz well and often to banish melancholy and irritability and bring peace and centering.

Comfort Food

This nourishing oil will deliver what ice cream can't.

20 drops grapefruit essential oil (*Citrus paradisi*) for healing, protection, self-esteem, renewal

30 drops benzoin essential oil (*Styrax tonkinensis*) for harmony, calm, love, peace of mind

10 drops black pepper essential oil (*Piper nigrum*) for protection, courage, and to drive away evil

Mix all essential oils and diffuse 1 drop of synergy per 100 ml water. Add 2 to 3 drops synergy to an aroma locket and wear it for empowering comfort.

Jasmine

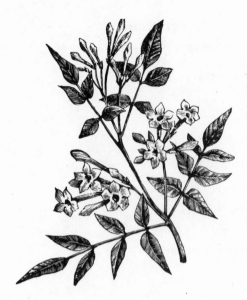

Scientific name: *Jasminum officinale*

Botanical family: Oleaceae

Origin: India, Morocco, France, Italy

Source of plant's oil: Flowers

Evaporation: Middle note

Scent description: Heady, thick floral; rich; sweet

Scent impact: Relieve anxiety, improve concentration

Magical Correspondences

Application: Diffuse, direct inhalation, dilute topically

Element: Water

Day: Monday

Magical uses: Love, lust, happiness, dreams, prosperity, justice, rest

Planet: Moon

Astrological sign: Cancer

Suggested crystal: Calcite—ruled by Cancer: energy magnifier

Deity/spirit: Diana, Roman goddess of the hunt, the moon, nature

Warnings

Avoid during pregnancy. Use sparingly, and dilute it, as it can cause sensitized skin issues if used when oxidized. Store tightly capped.

Herbal Lore

Jasmine is one of the most easily recognized florals in the aromatic arena. Its pale blossoms open at night and are picked by hand to flavor everything from tea to rice. Jasmine green tea is a treasured drink where green tea leaves are picked and allowed to dry in gardens of night-blooming jasmine. The dried tea leaves are then packed with dried flowers to preserve the delicate taste of the flowers.

Traditionally used in a variety of love spells and oils, including "Come to Me" blends, this flower has a long history of use for love, lust, and sex. It has been associated with not only arousing lovers of both genders but also reversing erectile dysfunction.

Jasmine's associations with the night and goddesses of the moon, darkness, and night come from the botanical habit of blooming at night. This serves multiple purposes for the plant. By opening at night, the fragrant oils produced by the flower are preserved by the petals being closed during the heat of the day. Night-blooming flowers have their own pollinator insects: flies, moths, beetles, and other flying insects. (The European honeybees we most associate with pollination are only active during the day.)

With jasmine being largely solvent extracted, it is hard to come by. Trained night laborers must pick 3,600,000 jasmine flowers for 1 pound of jasmine absolute. Because of the labor-intensive harvesting process, the waste built into the system, and the costs associated with solvent extraction, a pound of jasmine absolute can cost nearly $5,000. If the flowers are damaged, they will not yield the quality of oil expected of them.

Due to the high cost of this precious oil, companies often dilute the essential oil. Ethical companies will list on the bottle "jasmine absolute in jojoba" or some variant thereof. Unless the cost on the bottle is upward of $1,000 for a half ounce, there stands a good chance that the oil is diluted.

Another way to easily determine whether the oil is a fragrance oil or an essential oil is the composition of the bottle. If the oil is in plastic, or if the oil is in a clear glass bottle, it is either a heavily diluted perfume oil or a fragrance oil. Dark glass protects the integrity of the oil, as ultraviolet light degrades essential oils rapidly. A knowledgeable company will protect its investment by using dark-colored glass. It is common to see brown glass bottles, but cobalt and green glass are also used. For the purposes of essential oils, the color of the glass does not matter; it is merely an aesthetic choice.

There is nothing wrong with ethically diluting a precious oil so that it may be available to a wider market. The problem comes when companies declare they do not dilute, or when they state they do not adulterate their oil if they do. Over the years, home business marketing companies have been caught diluting their essential oils after using marketing buzz words like "therapeutic grade." There is no overseeing body that grades essential oil. There is no certification process. For more information on this, see the section on quality testing essential oils.

USES

Place a tissue with a drop of jasmine essential oil on it inside a pillowcase to bring sweet and loving dreams.

Diffuse 1 drop of jasmine essential oil per 100 ml water anytime to bring happiness. It's also uplifting during workings for joy.

Jasmine is synonymous with attraction, love, lust, fertility, and beauty. Wear diluted jasmine essential oil to feel sexy, inspire lust in others, and be reminded of the beauty within. Be careful, though. With jasmine's dependability in the arena of love, lust, and sex, users must examine their ethical compass, as jasmine has a darker reputation for magic involving binding lovers to the magic worker.

As a result of the historically high cost of this valuable oil, the association between jasmine and money goes back centuries. Jasmine magic, with both the oil and the flowers, relates it to money, prosperity, material objects, and "the finer things in life." When it is time to be rewarded with the finer things, anoint a green candle with diluted jasmine oil and inscribe with either the desired material object or a dollar sign, and burn in a fireproof dish.

The costs associated with these posh petals mean that in historic practice only clergy and royalty could afford them. This makes jasmine an excellent aid to connect with spirituality and/or goddesses.

Goddesses of the moon are especially adept at hearing the siren's call of jasmine.

In view of the antianxiety properties of jasmine, it is a divine partner for rest and relaxation. If you're having trouble getting to sleep, diffuse 1 drop of jasmine absolute in 100 ml of water thirty minutes before bedtime. Remember, restlessness becomes a habit, so try to establish a healthy sleep routine.

Desire to learn a new skill, trade, or hobby? Jasmine is well suited to magic ruling abilities, imagination, inspiration, and creativity. Light a candle while diffusing a drop of jasmine absolute and meditate, pray, journal, or plan how to go about learning that new skill.

Feeling a bit thin and worn out? Jasmine can patch any potential holes in your aura and help restore balance and wholeness to the self.

Astral projection is an intuitive skill that requires practice. That being said, working while diffusing jasmine absolute will yield a practiced effect more quickly than without.

When clarity is needed, it is often needed in a hurry. Diffuse jasmine absolute and meditate in a quiet space on the problem or question. For those adept in scrying, consider water scrying with a drop of jasmine absolute on top of the water in the dish. The aroma will still waft gently from the bowl and help with the clarity needed.

New ritual tools and spaces should be consecrated before use, and jasmine is just the flower for the job. A helping spirit for jasmine's consecration duties would be lavender and its properties. Fill a 10 ml bottle halfway with carrier oil, and add 1 drop jasmine absolute and 5 drops lavender essential oil for a powerful consecration oil that is easy on the senses and the wallet.

With connections to consecration and spirituality, it should come as no surprise that jasmine also works like magic for calming and centering energies. If there is adequate time and place for calming reflection, diffuse jasmine in water. If trying to attain calm under pressure and time constraints, direct inhalation from the bottle is possible, but a drop on a tissue is more likely to be beneficial and not overwhelm the senses. But use caution: direct inhalation with too much force, or without ventilation breaths, can lead to dizziness.

Though jasmine should be avoided during pregnancy, it has been used in magic and in practice to calm and soothe mothers-to-be during childbirth. Consult a care team if this seems beneficial to your birth plan. Alternatively, give the mom-to-be a small muslin bag with jasmine flowers in it to help ease the tensions of childbirth.

Disagreements can linger in the air, like last night's garlic. To clear the air after a disagreement, diffuse jasmine absolute. Who knows, maybe it will lead to making up.

Jasmine is a capable ally when used for defensive magic and protection. Mix 1 cup of rubbing alcohol with 3 drops jasmine absolute and sprinkle it around your home and property to create a defensive barrier.

Looking for an essential oil partner for divination purposes? Jasmine is just the one. Not only is it solid as a rock in the psychic department, but it is also calming and reduces anxiety around reading—truly a multifaceted ally.

If you are in the market for new friends and interesting acquaintances, jasmine can help fortify the friendliness factor. A single drop of jasmine essential oil in 10 ml carrier oil won't irritate the skin or overwhelm potential new friends. Make sure to get out there and try it! The magic cannot work if not given the proper chance. Join local groups, find folks with similar interests, and make introductions all around. It doesn't hurt that jasmine also boosts grace, harmony, and happiness.

Healing with jasmine is a gentle massaging away of pain and illness. Fill a small muslin bag with dried jasmine flowers and place a drop of jasmine essential oil in the bag. It will calm and soothe the person in need of healing and gently set them on the road to recovery.

Purification and uncrossing are some of the lesser-known associations of jasmine. Take a cup of grain-neutral spirits (vodka, moonshine, etc.) or rubbing alcohol and add 3 drops of jasmine absolute. Stir and sprinkle the mixture around the space with your hands, herbs, or branches.

Justice

Create justice, lift spirits, and protect with this blend.

2 drops jasmine absolute (*Jasminum officinale*) for justice, ability, clarity

3 drops benzoin essential oil (*Styrax tonkinensis*) for healing exorcism, hex breaking

15 drops frankincense essential oil (*Boswellia carteri*) for justice, banishing, protection

2 drops peppermint essential oil (*Mentha piperita*) for justice, good luck

Mix all oils and diffuse 1 drop synergy in 100 ml water during workings calling for justice. For an anointing oil, dilute 1 drop of synergy in 2 ml carrier oil. Add a pinch of coltsfoot (*Tussilago farfara*) to the anointing oil container before adding carrier to improve efficacy. Use the blend to anoint candles and charms for court cases, police involvement, justice work, hex breaking, and empowerment.

Court Magic

If the justice called for involves court, listen up. It is an old custom that names and birthdates carry the essence of a person. In the same vein, court cases have a true name and a birthdate. The true name of a court case could be the docket number, the file number, or even the name of the case (e.g., Jones v. Jones, State of California v. Jones, Jones v. Evil, Inc.). The birthdate would be the date on which the case was filed. Those pieces of information will be on official correspondence. The court case can be empowered or discreated by focusing on those pieces of information. A suggested working could involve making a copy of a letter from the court (originals may be needed in the case of hiring an attorney), anointing a white candle for purity or a black candle to banish the court case, and placing the candle in a fireproof dish. Anoint the copy of the letter with Justice Oil. See the Just Judge working on page 216 for additional help. Burn the banishing candle on a Saturday or the empowering candle on a Sunday and keep the letter on your altar or in a safe place until the case is settled.

Baby Blessing

Make this blend to use during the blessing of a newborn and wiccanings.

13 drops frankincense essential oil (*Boswellia carteri*) to bless and protect newborns

2 drops jasmine absolute for spiritual love, happiness, prosperity

2 drops May Chang essential oil (*Litsea cubeba*) for prayer, calm, strength

Diffuse this blend in the space where the blessing will take place. Mix all oils and add one drop synergy to a 2 ml bottle of the carrier oil of choice. Anoint the candles to be used during the ceremony.

Note: Do not apply essential oils to newborn skin, even if they are heavily diluted. It can cause burns and liver damage.

Lavender

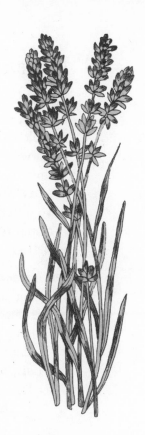

Scientific name: *Lavandula angustifolia*

Botanical family: Lamiaceae

Origin: France, Bulgaria, England, United States

Source of plant's oil: Flowers

Evaporation: Middle note

Scent description: Camphoraceous, sweet, floral

Scent impact: Restore balance, achieve calmness

Magical Correspondences

Application: Direct inhalation, diffusing, topical (neat or diluted)

Element: Air

Day: Wednesday

Magical uses: Sleep, antianxiety, protection, purification, centering, divination

Planet: Mercury

Astrological sign: Gemini, Virgo

Suggested crystal: Prehnite—ruled by Libra: facilitates meditation and visualization

Deities/spirits: Mercury, Roman god of financial gain, commerce, communication; Hecate, Greek goddess of magic and ghosts

Warnings

Use caution for pregnant women, children, and the elderly.

Herbal Lore

Lavender essential oil is so popular that when people say "aromatherapy," the first oil that comes to mind is usually lavender. Most notable in magical communities for use in dream pillows, this herb has a wide variety of uses and should not be underestimated simply because it is a popular and readily available plant.

Lavender has many faces; and while different types of lavender have differing uses in aromatherapy, all are treated the same when it comes to magical properties. Following are some of the lavender varieties you may come across:

- *Lavandula angustifolia* (true lavender) is one of the most popular essential oils on the planet, the Swiss Army knife of aromatherapists, who use it to treat everything from burns and insect bites to allergies and acne. This variety of lavender is sedating and is listed for antianxiety, sleeplessness, and more. *Lavandula officinalis* is nearly identical to this variety (though a less robust plant). The two species can be and are used interchangeably in all regards.

- *Lavandula spika* (spike lavender) is used frequently in respiratory ailments and infections. This variety has stimulating qualities for the mind.

- *Lavandula stoechas* (French lavender, lavender extra) is used in aromatherapy for sore muscles and aches and pains, as it has analgesic properties.

- *Lavandula x intermedia* (Lavendin) is a hybrid of L. spika and L. angustifolia. It has a citrus note and has also been called green lavender. It is more antiseptic than its parental varieties and has been used as a hospital disinfectant throughout Europe. Since lavendin produces more quickly than the parent varietals, it is cheaper than true lavender essential oil and is used in perfumes and cosmetics more often than lavender.

Lavender is associated with healing burns. The first recorded use of lavender essential oil being applied to a burn happened during a distillation of lavender oil. René-Maurice Gattefossé was burned, then splashed with lavender oil. He was stunned at how rapidly the burn healed.

Lavender has a reputation for banishing the evil eye in antiquity and is still used to purify spaces to this day. Burning the dried flowers on incense charcoal—or burning fresh lavender stems—is used to cleanse spaces and purify religous participants, and lavender is also useful for inducing sleep or a meditative state.

The reputation of lavender and love spells goes back to the height of Rome and its culture. Lavender and love are so intertwined that in Victorian England ladies of the night would anoint themselves in lavender perfume to attract customers and announce their profession. In the language of the Victorian Flower Oracle, lavender means "I am devoted to you." Use lavender in your magic to ask the gods to bring you a lover who is a devoted and loving partner.

USES

Lavender is one of the few essential oils that is nearly universally okayed for neat or undiluted application to the skin, except in pregnant women and young children.

Place a drop of lavender oil on a tissue and place inside a pillowcase to defeat anxiety that creeps in at bedtime. Alternately, fill a muslin tea bag with dried lavender flowers and place one drop of lavender essential oil on the bag before tucking into the pillowcase. It will last longer.

Diffuse one drop of lavender essential oil in water to ease the pain of grief or sorrow.

Lavender makes a helpful study aid, whether you're poring over dusty grimoires or textbooks alone or with a group. Increase your focus by diffusing lavender during study breaks, and take a tissue with a drop of lavender on it to gently inhale while taking the test.

Add a few drops of lavender essential oil to a tablespoon of salt, then mix into a spray bottle of water. This linen spray will encourage feelings of love, safety, and security. This will also make a gentle bug repellant to keep flying insects away from you in the great outdoors.

Add 3 drops of lavender essential oil to fountain pen ink for writing love letters.

One drop each of lavender essential oil and peppermint essential oil on a tissue can help release tensions that cause stress headaches.

To make romantic encounters more satisfying for committed partners, place 2 drops of lavender and 1 drop of rose absolute on blotting paper and place under the bed. The lavender takes the pressure off and encourages feelings of comfort and fidelity, while rose reminds the pair of attraction and romance.

House Blessing

Lavender is so ideally suited to purification it makes the perfect house blessing ingredient. Scrub your new pad and paint the walls if you choose. (Some folks even add essential oils to their wall paints to cut the smell during drying time.) Start either at the room farthest from the front door or at the hearth of the home—this can be a literal hearth or the kitchen stove. Burning an incense that is one part lavender and one part frankincense will cleanse and purify the home before you move in any furniture or belongings. Work your way around the dwelling, ending at the front door so anything nasty has a place to exit.

DIY Facial Toner

Herbal toners can be created at home, just like tinctures. Lavender toner is easy to make and is great for the skin as well. Place 2 teaspoons of dried lavender into 1 cup of apple cider vinegar. Bottle and keep in a dark cabinet for six weeks. Before using, add 1 cup of water or lavender hydrosol to the toner and apply with a cotton ball to refresh skin after cleansing. This is suitable for gift giving as well—just don't forget a decorative label! Tie a lavender stem to the bottom to remind the recipient what "flavor" it is. Other favorable combinations for facial toner include calendula, rosemary, thyme, chamomile, rose, and dried orange peel.

Health and Wellness Soak

Add desired amount of this bath salt to warm bathwater when a healing boost is needed.

10 drops lavender essential oil (*Lavandula angustifolia*) for
healing; antispasmodic

5 drops Roman chamomile essential oil (*Chameamelum
nobile*) for purification, curse breaking, sleep

1 drop lemongrass essential oil (*Cymbopogon citratus*) for
purification, soothing sore muscles

1 cup salt

Stir essential oils into the salt and sprinkle the mixture into warm
bathwater until desired scent is achieved. If you are well enough,
visualize your body hale and healthy during the bath.

Divine Light Protection Oil

Use when feeling particularly vulnerable.

10 drops lavender essential oil (*Lavandula angustifolia*) for
protection

6 drops frankincense (*Boswellia carterii*) for protection

8 drops steam-distilled Persian lime essential oil (*Citrus
latifolia*) for protection

Combine the essential oils and diffuse for divine protection. Alternately,
add 2 drops of synergy to a 10 ml roller bottle and fill with carrier oil.

Beltane Blessings Anointing Oil

Celebrate the Celtic May Day festival with this blend.

5 drops lavender essential oil (*Lavandula angustifolia*) for
love, health, peace

5 drops patchouli essential oil (*Pogostemon cablin*) for energy,
sex, aphrodisiac, grounding

5 drops tangerine essential oil (*Citrus reticulata*) for physical
energy, joy, purification

¼ cup carrier oil

Blend all essential oils in a glass or nonreactive bowl. Add carrier oil, and mix well. Store in a glass bottle.

Use to bless and purify anyone entering sacred space who is not allergic to any of the ingredients. Use with care, and print a copy of the ingredients to have on hand in case of allergy. Tangerine essential oil is reported to be non-phototoxic but can still present sensitivity issues in some. Use with care.

Thrice Purified

Blend three strong purification oils to banish the nasties.

> 5 drops lavender essential oil (*Lavandula angustifolia*)
> for purification
>
> 4 drops frankincense essential oil (*Boswellia carterii*)
> for purification
>
> 1 drop peppermint essential oil (*Mentha piperita*)
> for purification

Diffuse 1 drop synergy per 100 ml water to purify spaces. Alternatively, add 10 drops synergy to 8 teaspoons carrier oil to anoint people, places (homes and businesses), and objects that need purifying.

Meditation Oil

Use this blend to create a meditative state of mind.

> 2 drops lavender essential oil (*Lavandula angustifolia*)
> for peace
>
> 2 drops clary sage oil (*Salvia sclarea*) for psychic ability
>
> 1 drops patchouli oil (*Pogostemon cablin*) for grounding

Diffuse 1 drop synergy per 100 ml water to purify spaces. Alternatively, add 5 drops synergy to 4 teaspoons carrier oil to anoint pulse points (sides of the neck, wrists, and backs of knees) for peaceful meditation practice.

Lemon

Scientific name: *Citrus limon*

Botanical family: Rutaceae

Origin: Italy, United States

Source of plant's oil: Peels

Evaporation: Top note

Scent description: Bright, fresh, clean, sweet

Scent impact: Restore clear thinking, energize yourself and others

Magical Correspondences

Application: Direct inhalation, diffuse

Element: Water

Day: Monday

Magical uses: Clarity, calming, friendship, love, purification

Planet: Moon

Astrological sign: Cancer

Suggested crystal: Golden topaz—ruled by Sagittarius: stores energy and emotions

Deity/spirit: Philotes, Greek goddess of affection, friendship, and sex

Warnings

Cold-pressed lemon oil is phototoxic. Avoid direct sunlight on applied area for twelve to seventy-two hours, depending on sensitivity. Steam-distilled lemon essential oil is preferred for those who cannot avoid sunlight, as there are no phototoxic properties. Possible skin sensitizer.

Herbal Lore

It takes over 1,300 lemons to make one pound of lemon essential oil.

Uses

Diffuse 1 drop of lemon essential oil in 100 ml water to calm nervous agitation.

Diffuse lemon essential oil while meditating to gain clarity on an issue.

All citrus oils contain enough acid to act as a small battery—and this charge works in magic, too. Lemon increases the efficacy of spells by raising the power inherent in the charm or working. Add a drop of lemon essential oil to a mojo bag before sealing or dress the bag with a drop of lemon oil once a week to keep the power of the spell going.

Lemon is a steadfast ally in love spells, as it raises the vibrations of the magic worker to make them ready for new romantic relationships. Wear a drop of lemon oil in an aroma locket to signal to the universe your readiness for a new romantic partner.

The high and clear scent of lemon clears away the cobwebs of the mind and makes room for clear and focused thinking. Diffusing or directly inhaling lemon essential oil can provide mental clarity quickly.

Need a quick pick-me-up? Banish fatigue with a quick breath of lemon oil. A drop of lemon oil on a tissue or cotton ball, or even a gentle smell directly from the bottle, will help power through and get the job done. Remember, aromatherapy is helpful, but it's no replacement for sleep.

Diffuse a drop of lemon essential oil in 100 ml of water to purify a space of negative intentions or emotions.

A diluted, steam-distilled lemon essential oil will benefit professionals whose career requires emotional detachment. Police, therapists, nurses, funeral directors, and the like are in danger of bringing home the emotional baggage of others and will greatly benefit from having lemon essential oil as a perfume, scent blocker, and emotional-detachment enhancer. There are some professions where bringing home the emotions of others is potentially lethal. For those, remember: self-care is life care, and talk therapy is beneficial.

Concerned a lover may roam? Magical use of lemon can improve the mood of a partner, remind them of their initial attraction, and keep them faithful.

If you are in the market for new friends and interesting acquaintances, lemon eases loneliness and increases action, confidence, ability, and happiness. Diffuse while making plans for groups to join.

Working magic for abundance with lemon is a snap. One drop of lemon essential oil in 10 ml of carrier oil is low enough dilution to not irritate the skin, but make sure it is steam-distilled if venturing outside. Inscribe a dollar symbol ($) on a gold candle and burn on a Sunday.

Interested in working with the fae? Lemon is a bright oil that can help in contacting the faerie folk. Just remember they are not the glitter queens that popular culture might have people believe. Work with care, and do not say, "Thank you." It is considered offensive to the fair ones.

The acid inherent in citrus oils makes them prime allies for banishing diseases. Diffuse lemon in the sickroom, and use the anointing oil recipe mentioned above to anoint candles and pray for release from the disease. The magic of banishing should be undertaken under a waning moon if possible (though we all know that diseases wait for no lunar cycle). Sunday is an astrologically sound time to work.

Water scrying with essential oils is a potent scrying method. Fill a dark glass or stone bowl with water and add a single drop of lemon essential oil. Lemon allies get right down to business without the flowery language of actual flowers. For more in-depth answers, combine elements of air and water by scrying with a water diffuser. Watching these streams of steam emitted by a water diffuser can be very meditative and trance-inducing. Watch with an unfocused gaze and wait for the answers to come. It does not hurt that lemon is also

Cold pressed or distilled?

Here's a quick test to determine if the oil you're using was derived using distillation or cold pressed: Put a drop of the essential oil on a white index card. If the oil is brightly colored, it is likely cold pressed. If the oil is clear, it is likely steam-distilled. Dilute and give a patch test before venturing into direct sun. No magical working is worth a blistering burn.

associated with water magic and spirit guides. (For more information on scrying, see the section on divination at the end of this book.)

The opposite side of that coin is the increased focus that lemon brings. It is such a sharp note with a high vibration that it gets right to the heart of the matter. When focus is paramount, give a gentle sniff from the bottle or carry a tissue with a drop of oil on it. It will help zero in the focus with laser precision.

Diffuse lemon essential oil in your home or office to increase joy and happiness and remind yourself to lighten up. These qualities, including stress relief, also make lemon a great partner for love magic.

Longevity and lemon go hand in hand. Lemon essential oil can prolong the competence of magical workings, as it keeps going long after some of the more gentle fragrances have petered out. Speaking of which, it also has a reputation for magic involving more physical forms of longevity.

To increase openness, there is no plant better suited than lemon. It dissipates depression as well as enhances joy and love. Lemon opens the soul and lets out the cobwebs and moths, and fills the heart space with light and laughter. Even the energetic spaces can use a bit of spring cleaning every once in a while. Take time to breathe the scent of lemon and meditate on ways to connect with the person you want to be.

Lemon can increase the security of home and property. Dried lemon peel scented with a drop of lemon essential oil can create a well-lit boundary when placed around the property. Lemon's connection with divination can also be focused to alert the magic worker to anyone testing the wards of the home.

Lemon is an incredible therapeutic ally for working through and releasing trauma. Lemon is uplifting and can bolster our inner defenses while we examine and work through the hurtful things, and let go of our past.

Spring Cleaning

Use this blend for an emotional clearing out.

2 drops lemon essential oil (*Citrus limon*) for clarity, blessing, purification, focus

1 drop ginger essential oil (*Zingiber officinale*) to energize and bring luck, improvement, inspiration

4 drops petitgrain essential oil (*Citrus aurantium*) to banish depression, increase physical energy, joy, purification

Diffuse this blend when the emotional cobwebs need to be swept out. Place one drop in 100 ml of water in diffuser. Place 1 drop in 2 ml of carrier oil for anointing candles. If you plan to apply the oil, use steam-distilled lemon essential oil and dilute 2 drops in a 10 ml bottle filled with carrier oil. The scent will be light, but should not sensitize skin.

Deep Breaths

This blend is protective, calming, and balancing.

1 drop steam-distilled lemon essential oil (*Citrus limon*) for releasing trauma, lifting depression, banishing fatigue, balancing

1 drop lavender (*Lavandula angustifolia*) for calm, harmony, secrets

3 drops sandalwood (*Santalum album*) for protection, harmony, calm

Diffuse this blend to bolster those defenses, release painful secrets, and empower the entire self with calming harmony. Secrets are toxic; use this oil to empower the self and let them go.

Five drops in a 10 ml bottle with carrier oil will be a low enough dilution for anointing candles, charms, and bags. Anoint photos to release their connection.

Write secrets on flash paper and burn them. They will go in a flash of light, destroying any hold they have. Flash paper leaves no smoke, ash, or burned paper bits behind, and the secrets can be left out as well, peacefully. The next step is to make sure anyone affected by the secret is also safe and secure. Even if we release our attachments to them, they can still affect others.

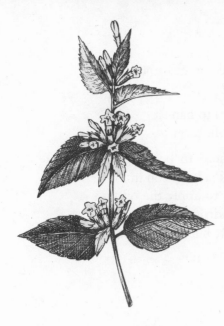

Lemon Balm (aka Melissa)

Scientific name: *Melissa officinalis*

Botanical family: Lamiaceae

Origin: France, Utah

Source of plant's oil: Flowers

Evaporation: Middle note

Scent description: Citrusy, sweet, clean, fresh

Scent impact: Encourage a gentle nature, soothe what ails you

Magical Correspondences

Application: Topical with low dilution, diffuser, direct inhalation

Element: Water

Day: Monday

Magical uses: Healing, success, love, calm, fertility, soothing, connecting with the Goddess

Planet: Moon

Astrological sign: Cancer

Suggested crystal: White opal—ruled by Libra: stimulates self-esteem

Deity/spirit: Hecate, Greek goddess of witchcraft, and ghosts

Warnings

Use in a low dilution for possible skin sensitizing properties.

Herbal Lore

It is so well known that bees prefer lemon balm that its Latin binomial, melissa, means honeybee. As bees are constantly working, lemon balm never stops working for the person wielding it.

The purifying qualities of the plant are so well known that this oil was even used to scent, and thereby purify, wooden furniture. The popular lemon-scented wood polishes and protectors derive their smell from this practice, and from the aromatic idea that lemon equals clean.

Keep in mind that although melissa is a prolific herb of the mint family, only the plant's small white blossoms are used to make this delicately scented oil. Due to the price of this highly prized sedative oil, it is very difficult to find melissa absent a carrier oil. Ethical companies diluting this precious oil to protect the wallets of consumers will clearly state on the label that the oil is diluted for the ease of use by the practitioner. See more about how to test the essential oils in the section on quality testing to make sure the oil has not been diluted with fillers or water.

Uses

Melissa is a gently scented essential oil of great use in healing magic. Aromatherapists suggest it to treat itching, irritation, fungal infections, and more.

As with any of the citrus-scented essential oils, melissa is used in magic for success, business acumen, and wealth. When starting a new business venture, prepare a candle with melissa anointing oil (1 drop melissa in 10 ml carrier oil) before burning.

Lemon balm is uplifting and encourages happiness in magic. Diffuse a drop of melissa essential oil in 100 ml water while making a list of joyful things, including anything that can and does bring joy. Keep that list for days that are harder, emotionally speaking.

For those trying to conceive, melissa is associated with fertility magic. Dried herb, fresh flowers, and lemon balm essential oil are all beneficial tools. If a figural candle of a baby is handy, all the better. Unadorned candles, such as tea lights, tapers, and chime candles, will also work. Simply anoint the candles with the low-dilution anointing oil described above. Writing something like "new baby" on the candle can also help the working. Burn the candle on a Friday or Monday for best results.

Melissa is an herb of compassion and comfort, and is well suited to those in hospice. Diffuse a drop or two of melissa essential oil in personal space to reduce grief and stave off compassion fatigue and sorrow. Melissa is especially adept at soothing emotional wounds.

With the lunar associations of lemon balm, it stands to reason that this oil is capable of reaching out to goddesses associated with the moon. Diffuse melissa essential oil, burn dried lemon balm on incense charcoal, or anoint the third eye and wrists with low-dilution lemon balm oil when seeking an audience with a goddess of the moon—particularly Artemis, Diana, or Selene—or Hecate, the Greek underworld goddess of night and witchcraft.

Love spells cast with melissa bring the correct partner, who is gentle, compassionate, and joyful. Anoint a red or pink candle while listing your ideal traits of a romantic partner. Remember, this is a love note to the self. Making a list so specific it infringes on another's free will is an ethical quandary, so tread carefully. To draw a new lover, add a sprig of lemon balm to a pocket.

Lemon balm is a capable sedative. For magic involving peace, banishing anxiety, grounding excitable emotions, and circular thinking, turn to melissa. It will help narrow focus in a positive and calming way. In addition, it banishes depression in a wholly satisfying way.

Looking to master a new skill? Lemon balm works with ordered thinking and increased focus to help determine the best course of action. The associations are also beneficial for practicing a newly acquired skill and engaging memory. It also lends itself to clarity of thought to cut through the newness confusion.

Along with helping build business acumen, melissa is known to bestow the benefits of good fortune on its user. Blessing new business spaces with melissa ensures a steady stream of customers. Diffuse melissa essential oil during business-planning sessions, anoint the doors of physical businesses, and thank the Lady of the Moon for her blessings.

To make effective magic, Melissa can be a constructive ally for learning to ground and center quickly and easily. Once these techniques are managed, magic becomes more effortless, and less about gut reactions.

Growth, both mental and emotional, is possible through work with lemon balm. It helps remove the ego from the equation and allows the development to take place with less effort. If there is a recognized area that needs work, diffuse lemon balm while making a list of ways to improve. If it is helpful, copy it into a journal, diary, or Book of Shadows. Then anoint a candle with diluted lemon balm and place the list under it. Burn the list after the candle burns out. (Remember, use fireproof dishes, and never leave a burning candle unattended. Fire safety is no joke.)

For those looking to unlock memories from a past life, melissa is the ally to seek out. It strips away the confines and illusions of time to create a safe and secure space for exploring those lives previously lived. Diffuse its essential oil during meditation to discover who you used to be.

Melissa can gently encourage the analysis of memories and emotional trauma that still have weight to them. Proceed gently, as memories often have sharp edges. Melissa can bolster feelings of anxiety, stress, and lack of grounding. Seeking out a licensed and trained therapist can be empowering. It helps with recovery from violence and trauma.

Trouble sleeping? Lemon balm is also used in magic for deep meditation. Diffusing lemon balm while meditating, practicing square or circular breathing (see below), and setting an intention for sleep are helpful ways to gently drift off. If sleeplessness becomes a habit, examine your sleep hygiene for a culprit before taking further steps.

The properties that allow melissa to benefit alleviate anxiety and depression also make it a boost for the sex life of committed partners' sex lives. It increases arousal responses in men and women, improves sociability, and enhances feelings of safety and security. Diffuse melissa essential oil for the best benefit.

If problems with headaches, diseases of the brain, or lack of focus are present, developing a relationship with lemon balm is a must.

Square and Circular Breathing

A key part of meditation is noticing your breath. Here are a couple different ways you can breathe consciously during your practice.

- Circular breath: slow and mindful breaths (sometimes counted) in and out without pause, usually in through the nose and out through the mouth.
- Square breath: a counted breath with four "sides." Start with a four-count breath in through the nose. Hold that breath for four counts. Release for four counts through the mouth. Hold the exhaled breath for a four count and repeat.

The magic in melissa brings a focus and acts as a talisman to ward off future problems. Anoint the candle of choice with lemon balm anointing oil and write a word or two on the candle to focus intent.

Know a youth in need of protection? Goddesses of the moon see all that happens in the dark and are particularly attuned to children. Petition the deity of choice for safety regarding that young person, anoint a candle for them, and let it burn. If the situation warrants it, consider police or other official intervention for the child or children in question. They will thank you when they are older.

Gold Galore

Good fortune awaits when you use this blend.

10 drops lemon balm essential oil (*Melissa officinalis*) for good fortune, success, joy, money

10 drops myrrh essential oil (*Commiphora myrrha*) for good luck, prosperity, transformation, success

1 drop peppermint essential oil (*Mentha piperita*) for good luck, happiness

5 drops petitgrain essential oil (*Citrus aurantium*) for purification, transformation, joy

Mix all oils, and place 1 drop synergy in a 2 ml bottle and fill with carrier oil for magical use. Unlike the fast cash and purifying financial past oils covered elsewhere in this book, this oil is designed to bestow luck, fortune, success, and happiness. Money cannot buy happiness, but it is easier to cry in a BMW than on a bike. This oil uses both myrrh and lemon balm, which are commonly sold in an already diluted form, so their drop-count will be higher than oils that are not diluted. Let your nose be your guide. The better it smells to you, the more likely you are to use it—and the likelier it is to work.

Lemongrass

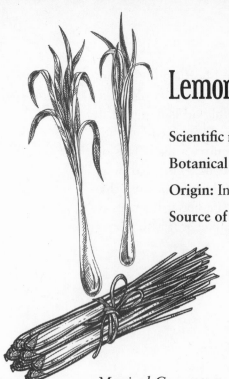

Scientific name: *Cymbopogon citratus*

Botanical family: Poaceae

Origin: India

Source of plant's oil: Leaves

Evaporation: Top note

Scent description: Clean, green, citrusy, and herbal

Scent impact: Cleanse your space, increase intuition

Magical Correspondences

Application: Direct inhalation, diffusion, topical with low dilution to prevent sensitization

Element: Air

Day: Wednesday

Magical uses: Fidelity, passion, protection, purification, intuition

Planet: Mercury

Astrological sign: Gemini

Suggested crystal: Amber—ruled by Leo: strength, courage of conviction, changing negative energy into positive

Deity/spirit: Airmed, Celtic goddess of healing

Warnings

Use in low dilution (under 2.5 percent), as skin irritation may occur. Do not use with young children, as it may irritate mucosal lining in nose and throat. Check for possible drug interactions.

Herbal Lore

Lemongrass is popular in Ayurvedic medicine and has been called "Indian melissa." It is used in Ayurvedic practice to cool fevers, relieve pain from inflammation, and reduce stress and anxiety.

Magical practitioners know that lemongrass is a potent ally for intuitive work, card reading, divination, scrying, and tea leaf reading. In hoodoo, lemongrass is used for deep cleansing and uncrossing work. It is one of the main ingredients in van van oil to remove obstacles, and floor washes to keep evil away. (Van van oil can be difficult to make due to material sourcing, but it is easily found in your local shop or online—see Appendix D: Botanical Magic Resources.) Dried lemongrass is commonly carried in a mojo bag to keep loved ones safe from physical harm.

As a member of the lemon-scented family, there will be some family resemblance between the uses of the lemon-scented herbs, even ones that are not featured in this book, like lemon-scented geranium.

Uses

Because lemongrass is such a dynamic partner in the realm of the psychic, it is a natural choice for psychic growth and development. Diffuse a drop of lemongrass essential oil in 100 ml water while meditating on methods to expand consciousness. Practice tarot, guided meditations, and astral travel.

Feeling worn down? Lemongrass is physically, emotionally, and spiritually refreshing. Wear the diluted oil on the pulse points, carry a tissue with a drop of essential oil on it, or add a drop of lemongrass to an aroma locket for a quick, refreshing pick-me-up. This uplifting oil will have you feeling like new in no time.

Looking to master a new skill or ability? Lemongrass is a Mercury-aligned herb and works with communication and ordered thinking as well as increased focus to help determine the best course of action. The associations are also beneficial for practicing a newly acquired skill and engaging memory. It also lends itself to clarity of thinking to cut through the newness confusion.

To quiet a racing mind, take a deep breath with lemongrass. It can help restore balance and encourage calm, improve concentration, and bring clarity.

Lemongrass's strong citrus scent cuts right to the chase and helps keep people honest. Diffuse its essential oil before having a difficult conversation if lies or half-truths may be invited to the table. Place one drop of lemongrass oil in 100 ml water in a diffuser up to thirty minutes before sitting down to talk.

Seeking a connection to the divine? Lemongrass bridges the worlds and can lead to a feeling of connection with Them. Diffuse while meditating on the nature of the Divine with whom the connection is sought.

With the uplifting scent of lemon, this member of the grass family makes reigniting the flames of passion a snap. Anoint a candle with one drop of lemongrass oil in a 10 ml bottle. Burn on a Friday to remind your partner what originally attracted them to you.

Place a drop of lemongrass essential oil on a tissue and put it inside your lover's pillowcase to keep them faithful.

Lemongrass has been planted around homes for hundreds of years to keep snakes away. This and its reputation for protection have helped earn it a reputation for protecting the home from wild animals. Snakes are a beautiful and beneficial part of the ecosystem, and there's no need to harm them if found on the property. Many snake species are harmless to humans and eat pests most would rather not deal with. Avoid the snake and it will avoid being seen in return. If a worrisome snake is spotted, call the local wildlife extension or wild animal rescue and follow their explicit instructions.

Lemongrass not only has a reputation for increasing psychic abilities, due to its airy and intellectual associations, but it is also responsible for expanding awareness outside the physical body. This lends itself to use in magical security for the self and home. The oil also has a standing in the realm of encouraging visions.

Lemongrass's sunny disposition makes it an ideal candidate for attracting goodness and good luck. Write a petition on flash paper detailing what luck is needed, and why. Anoint a gold or yellow candle with lemongrass anointing oil and burn it. As the flame begins to die, burn the flash paper to release your intention into the world.

For personal growth, lemongrass is well suited. It inflames passion and is still an herb of protection. It fans the flames of change and empowers honesty and good luck.

If the outside world has become too loud, lemongrass can provide solace, a quiet haven from the noise and needs of the exterior. Diffuse its essential oil during a quiet time for yourself. Turn your phone and the television off, and unless the radio is producing soothing music feel free to turn it off too. Silence is healing, and so is lemongrass.

The strength the plant and its fragrance mean it's valuable for work in physical strength, hex breaking, and uncrossing work. Sprinkle dried lemongrass around the home for uncrossing. Diffuse the oil when strength is needed for a physically exhausting task at hand.

Lie Detector

This blend is useful in ferreting out the truth.

- 2 drops lemongrass essential oil (*Cymbopogon citratus*) for honesty, increased awareness

- 2 drops myrrh essential oil (*Commiphora myrrha*) for protection, compassion

- 1 drop rosemary essential oil (*Rosmarinus officinalis*) for confidence, character, strength

Add 1 drop of synergy to 2 ml bottle of carrier oil. Shake well and anoint candle. Write topic of truth to be determined and burn. The truth will come out. Diffuse before difficult conversations where truth is needed.

Litha Lessons

Use this blend on the first day of summer to connect with the divine masculine.

- 10 drops lemongrass essential oil (*Cymbopogon citratus*) for a quiet mind, connection, psychic growth

- 8 drops cedarwood essential oil (*Cedrus atlantica*) for consecration, divination, strength

20 drops lavender essential oil (*Lavandula angustifolia*) for balance, calm, harmony, divination

Combine essential oils in a 2 ml bottle and diffuse on the first day of summer to celebrate the warming of the earth.

Battle Hexes

This is Sparta!

10 drops clary sage essential oil (*Salvia sclarea*) for centering, secrets, wisdom

15 drops fennel essential oil (*Foeniculum vulgare*) to battle hexes

15 drops lemongrass essential oil (*Cymbopogon citratus*) for physical energy, increased awareness, and improved mood

5 drops vetiver essential oil (*Vetiveria zizanioides*) to balance and seal the aura

Use this oil for offensive or defensive magic. Defensive magic is commendable, dissolving a nasty hex and grounding the hateful energy. But sometimes magic needs to be on the offense. This is an oil of action. This is a warning. An oil that says, "Leave me alone, or I will hit back."

Add 1 drop synergy to 2 ml carrier oil to use as anointing oil. Add 1 drop of synergy to 100 ml water diffuser to protect your home or space.

Quiet Voices Divination Oil

Use this blend for divination, centering, and solitude.

2 drops lemongrass essential oil (*Cymbopogon citratus*) for thought, intellect, connection, the Divine

2 drops rosemary essential oil (*Rosmarinus officinalis*) for release, strength, meditation

1 drop tangerine essential oil (*Citrus reticulate*) for divination, defensive magic, inspiration

Enjoy the quiet and the solitude. Find the person you are. Meet the person you should be. Useful for divination; quiet the to-do list, the worries, and the fears long enough to journey inward.

Mix all essential oils and diffuse 1 drop synergy per 100 ml water when an inner journey is needed or desired.

Magnet Oil

Draw the right loving partner.

1/8 ounce beeswax granules

1/8 ounce vanilla-infused jojoba oil

4 drops ginger essential oil (*Zingiber officinale*) for energizing, love, passion, strength, protection

3 drops lemongrass essential oil (*Cymbopogon citratus*) for passion, fidelity, honesty, uplifting

6 drops patchouli essential oil (*Pogostemon cablin*) for love, passion, protection, peace of mind, aphrodisiac

5 drops Turkish rose absolute (*Rosa damascene*) for love, luck, peace

Gently heat the beeswax in a double boiler until granules are melted. Quickly remove from heat and incorporate jojoba. Allow to cool slightly, stirring consistently. Add ginger, lemongrass, patchouli, and Turkish rose oils gradually while continuing to stir. Carefully pour into small pots (usually sold for lip balm) and apply to pulse points to attract the right partner. Note: This spell is a magnet; it will not impede the free will of another.

Synergy can also be used as an anointing oil for candles, charms, and talismans.

Steady Ground

Use this heavy-duty grounding oil in times of anxiety or fear, or when you are too busy to meditate.

2 drops balsam fir essential oil (*Abies balsamea*) for grounding, clarity

1 drop lemongrass essential oil (*Cymbopogon citratus*) to improve concentration, relieve anxiety

5 drops patchouli essential oil (*Pogostemon cablin*) for grounding, protection, increased power of spells

Mix all oils and diffuse synergy in ritual spaces, offices (where permitted), and homes when strong grounding is needed. It is even more important to meditate when we do not have time to do it.

Mandarin

See Tangerine.

Myrrh

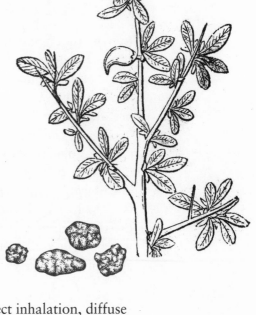

Scientific name: *Commiphora myrrha*

Botanical family: Burseraceae

Origin: Somalia

Source of plant's oil: Resin

Evaporation: Base note

Scent description: Dark, woody, earthy

Scent impact: Release negative emotions
and thought patterns

Magical Correspondences

Application: Topical with proper dilution, direct inhalation, diffuse

Element: Fire

Day: Tuesday

Magical uses: compassion, protection, hex breaking, happiness, luck

Planet: Mars

Astrological sign: Aries

Suggested crystal: Rhyolite—ruled by Sagittarius: fire of creation

Deity/spirit: Archangel Michael

Warnings

Women who are pregnant or breastfeeding should avoid myrrh. Do not use if you are diabetic, have a fever, or have a heart condition. Use with care during menses, as it increases menstrual flow.

Herbal Lore

Myrrh is a commonly heard though vastly misunderstood member of the family that also contains frankincense. These two resins are frequently conflated, and many people don't know that *Commiphora myrrha* is its own tree that provides resin in the same manner as its best friend, frankincense.

Young children are told the story of Jesus Christ being brought gifts of gold, frankincense, and myrrh. These gifts are repeated so often that even seasoned adults believe frankincense and myrrh are one object, "frankincense-and-myrrh."

The incredible display of wealth in gifting a baby items such as myrrh, gold, and frankincense is staggering, considering this child was born in a manger. Mary and Joseph would never need to work again if they merely sold the gifts bestowed upon their child.

Uses

The fire inherent in this solar plant resin makes it ideal for hex breaking, endings, and transformation work. When it's time for things to die—bad habits, unhealthy relationships, and curses—burn myrrh resin, diffuse quality myrrh essential oil, or anoint a candle with diluted myrrh oil (estimating a 10 percent dilution that many essential oil companies use, 3 drops in a 10 ml bottle would give a 2.5 percent dilution).

Wealth and prosperity are within reach with myrrh. To gain material objects, myrrh is beneficial. The solar aspects of the oil garner favor for prosperity, gratitude, success, and progress. Here's a simple ritual for prosperity using myrrh: Copy one side of the highest denomination bill you can get your hands on. Cut it out to bill size, and write your material goal (e.g., "new house," "startup capital for my small business," etc.) on the back. Place a drop of myrrh oil on the paper, and anoint the candle with diluted myrrh oil before burning.

Myrrh is one of the ultimate comforting scents, especially for anyone with an ecclesiastical background, particularly Orthodox Christians and Catholics. Myrrh is associated with happiness and growth. Diffusing this oil when times are emotionally trying, when we are feeling particularly fragile, or when we are simply in need of ardent support is soothing and comforting.

Myrrh is used to heal emotional pain and bring peace and wash away sorrow. To make myrrh spray, add 3 drops myrrh essential oil to 1 tablespoon witch haze in a 2-ounce spray bottle. Fill with water and shake to mix. Mist around body when comfort is needed.

Since myrrh is linked with meditation, it is a natural go-to for a calming influence. When feeling the desire to be calm or centered, turn to myrrh. Anoint the third eye and the wrist pulse points or diffuse 1 drop of myrrh essential oil in 100 ml water.

Consecration with myrrh was popular even before its numerous mentions in the Bible. While myrrh's astrological correspondences are solar, it is also associated with lunar mysteries and goddesses of the night. Many types of sacred duties were performed by this resin. Before going out for a night of lunar revelry, anoint the third eye (the center of the forehead) with diluted myrrh oil for consecration, happiness, power, and protection.

Myrrh is a healing, restorative resin. It was one of the first medicines in recorded history. Even well-known, reputable scientific websites discuss medical uses for myrrh. It can be a balm for the aura, bringing healing and restoring a healthy aura. Meditate while diffusing myrrh essential oil and see the self as a whole, with a secure and balanced aura. Myrrh is also understood to be an oil and a resin that is capable of stimulating the chakras if there is an energetic blockage. It will also bring those solar associations to the healing of the self with strength and warmth.

Myrrh is associated with astral as well as physical strength. Anoint the pulse points inside each elbow or wrist with diluted myrrh oil when strength is needed.

The sacred nature of the myrrh resin and its essential oil brings honor and manifests desires. If there is a desire to serve others with honor, whether through the military, law enforcement, or another first responder capacity, anoint a candle and outline honorable intentions on a sheet of paper. Place the paper under the candle while it burns.

The numinous nature of myrrh also lends itself to counteracting evil. It can destroy illnesses that are the result of a hex and restore virility.

Myrrh helps to release. It helps to banish bitterness and discord, especially in romantic relationships. It allows calm and rational discourse. If a relationship is coming to an end, myrrh can help resolve things safely and rationally for all, while helping everyone through the grief process, resulting in growth for all parties involved.

The light of the sun shines on unions created under myrrh's energies. To create a lasting and loving harmony, use myrrh to ask the gods for the perfect romantic partner. Write the qualities of the perfect romantic partner and place them under a candle anointed with diluted myrrh oil on a Friday or anytime during the waxing to full lunar phase. Myrrh will also give you the confidence to go out and meet the perfect person.

Myrrh oil is associated with the blessing of babies. Simply diffuse myrrh oil in the space where the baby blessing, wiccaning, or other ritual is performed.

If negative experiences can potentially be attributed to spirits, myrrh is a powerful helper for exorcism work. It will shine the light of the Divine and banish negativity, and is uncrossing, making the affected space inhospitable to further mucking about. Myrrh transforms the vibes of a place without leaving it open to new spirit disturbances.

Myrrh oil carries with it the calm and emotional tranquility that can be had at the altar of the religion of choice. The warmth inherent in spiritual fulfillment is held within the resin as well as the oil. Burn the resin, diffuse the oil in a water diffuser, or anoint pulse points with diluted myrrh oil.

To quickly and easily add power to mojo bags, place a myrrh tear (a drop of hardened resin that forms during harvesting) inside. It does not need to be a large piece. Myrrh and other resins act like magical batteries, powering the magic over the long term. If myrrh tears are not available, simply place a drop of myrrh essential oil on the bag once a week.

As in the tarot, everything the light touches is golden. Success can be had, and good luck is on your side. With myrrh, luck and success are just a drop away. Open blockages to prosperity and luck with this determined aide.

Wondering if past-life baggage could be responsible for current conflicts? Myrrh's meditative qualities can aid past-life recall. Burn myrrh resin while meditating on the lives led before now. Water scrying is possible with either a bowl of water and a drop of myrrh oil or a drop of myrrh oil in a water diffuser.

Being the strongest of the plant allies, resins are particularly well suited to protection and grounding work—they have the patience of the trees from which they originate. Burn myrrh resin in the home to protect it. Add a drop of myrrh essential oil to an aroma locket to protect the person wearing it. Protect passengers as well as the conveyance by placing myrrh inside the car. Do not let it overheat, though, as the resin could melt. Placing it in an unused ashtray, change well, or muslin bag in the glove box should prevent it from causing any damage should it melt. Car diffusers are also gaining popularity.

Purification is the hallmark of any resin, but most assuredly ones that have a history of use in churches and other places of worship. Frankincense, copal, and myrrh come immediately to mind. Diffuse the essential oil to purify and enliven space. Burn the resin where able to purify spaces of negativity, sadness, and ill intent.

Mercy

Use this blend to grant forgiveness and release emotional burdens, even to one's self.

   1 drop myrrh essential oil (*Commiphora myrrha*) for
      compassion, relieving feelings of grief

   1 drop lemon balm (*Melissa officinalis*) for fostering calm
      and compassion, and releasing grief

   1 drop neroli essential oil (*Citrus aurantium*) for releasing
      negative emotions

Lemon balm, myrrh, and neroli are used to grant forgiveness and release emotional burdens. This oil is comprised of three of the most common commercially diluted essential oils on the market. Start with an even ratio as you mix the oils, and adjust based on scent and your preference. If the oil is of a superior quality, less is needed.

Diffuse or mix with carrier oil and apply to pulse points.

Neroli
(aka Bitter Orange)

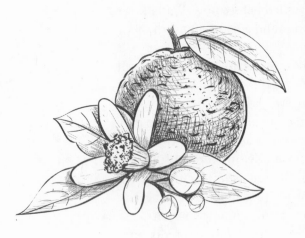

Scientific name: *Citrus aurantium*

Botanical family: Rutaceae

Origin: Morocco

Source of plant's oil: Flowers

Evaporation: Top note

Scent description: Citrusy, sweet, lightly floral

Scent impact: Fight depression, bring peace

Magical Correspondences

Application: Diffuse, dilute, direct inhalation

Element: Fire

Day: Sunday

Magical uses: Purification, confidence, joy, protection, sleep

Planet: Sun

Astrological sign: Leo

Suggested crystal: Sunstone—ruled by Leo: banishes fear

Deity/spirit: Guan Yu, Taoist god of brotherhood and righteousness (in the context of war)

Warnings

Dilute or use sparingly. Headaches can result from using too much of this oil.

Herbal Lore

Neroli oil is derived from the flowers of the bitter orange tree (*Citrus aurantium*). Petitgrain and bitter orange are also included herein because they all come from *Citrus aurantium* and would have the same magical uses. Rather than duplicate the magical materials, the sections were merged under the most popular of the three oils.

Neroli was introduced to the Mediterranean region when Arab traders brought it there from China. The cost of bringing this precious oil either through the South China Sea or across India meant that for many years it was only available to royalty and the ultrarich. Due to the extreme cost of the oil, the flowers rather than oil were used in wedding ceremonies. Orange blossoms are traditionally associated with Hera and Juno as they were placed in bridal bouquets to calm pre-wedding jitters. Brides were also anointed with orange blossom waters to ask Hera or Juno to bless the union with fertility and happiness.

Neroli is the essential oil derived from the flowers of the bitter orange tree (*Citrus aurantium*). Three essential oils are derived from the bitter orange tree: bitter orange oil is steam distilled from the peel; neroli oil is solvent extracted from the flowers; and petitgrain oil, a middle note oil, is distilled from the stems and leaves. Since all three essential oils derive from the same tree, and neroli can be cost-prohibitive, it is common for botanical magic practitioners to substitute bitter orange or petitgrain oil for neroli oil in magic. Please bear in mind the differences in phototoxicity and scent profiles between the oils:

Cold-pressed bitter orange essential oil is phototoxic.

Petitgrain is not phototoxic; nor is steam-distilled bitter orange.

Instead of a top note, petitgrain is a middle note and should be blended accordingly.

Since bitter orange is derived from the rind of the bitter orange fruit (not to be confused with *Citrus sinensis*, the sweet orange), it will be cheaper than petitgrain, which is likely cheaper than neroli. Plan accordingly.

Neroli is on the list of the most commonly diluted and chemically adulterated oils. Beware of "neroli oil" that is sold in clear glass bottles, that seems unreasonably cheap, or that is clear in color.

USES

The solar associations of the citrus family make it well suited to protection work. The shielding aspects mean that it will stand up under heavy fire and even works on psychic attacks. Diffuse neroli essential oil in the home if you fear an attack directed at either your home or someone residing inside. If a specific threat is understood, anoint the subject with diluted neroli oil (3 drops neroli essential oil in a 10 ml roller bottle filled with carrier) and anoint the intended target. Prayers are also acceptable, if desired, but not required.

Since calming neroli and soothing petitgrain essential oils work as a sedative, they are perfect allies for magic involving sleep and stress relief, since these often go hand in hand. Place a tissue with a drop of neroli essential oil inside your pillowcase to induce sleep. For magic involving stress relief, diffuse a drop of the essential oil in a 100 ml water diffuser.

Neroli is one of the most beneficial antianxiety essential oils out there. It encourages the release of negative emotions. Because of the magical association of release and uplifting, it is well suited to help reduce the impact of sexual trauma, especially when used in conjunction with talk therapy with a licensed therapist. The antianxiety effect is markedly noted in the petitgrain essential oil as well.

With neroli's matrimonial associations, the fertility aspect can sometimes be overshadowed. If you desire a new addition to the family, or a more fertile environment for your small business or project, anoint a green candle with diluted neroli oil. (See chapter 2 for more candle color information.) Write your intention on a piece of paper and place it underneath the candleholder. Light the candle (in a fireproof container; never leave a burning candle unattended) and state your intent out loud. Burn during the waxing portion of the month, or on a Friday.

Work with neroli or petitgrain can help increase both the psychic senses and physical awareness. Because of this, neroli makes an incredible addition to protection and hex-breaking blends. It serves to alert the person monitoring the wards of a home or business that someone is attempting to cause trouble. To head an issue off at the pass, write your intention on a piece of paper and place it underneath the candleholder. Light the candle (in a fireproof container; never leave a burning candle unattended) and state your intent out loud. Burn during the waning portion of the month, or on a Sunday. A black candle is suggested, but as they can be hard to come by, feel free to substitute the color that feels correct.

Change is a large part of the human condition, because that which does not change inevitably dies. If change occurs suddenly, or is too close to home, grief is only natural. Neroli can help process grief in a beneficial way. If grief is impacting day-to-day life after a significant period of time, remember there is help available.

Neroli and petitgrain are excellent herbal allies for establishing and nurturing self-confidence. They are uplifting oils and help act as emotional scaffolding while the structure is strengthened. If emotional support is needed, anoint the wrists and behind the ears with diluted neroli oil, or add a drop to an aroma locket until strength is restored.

Neroli and petitgrain are both entrusted with magic reserved for banishing depression. With depression can come physical sensitivity to certain pressures. Neroli can help with both of these conditions. Anoint a figural candle in a color associated with healing (pink, green, pale blue), and name it for the person experiencing pain and depression. Burn on a Sunday.

Citrus scents as well as florals are associated with joy and happiness. If a little joy is needed, diffuse neroli essential oil in the home or office or add to an aroma locket for an extra spring in your step.

Neroli is not just orange's sleepy cousin. It is an excellent collaborator for guided journeys and meditation of all kinds. Diffuse its essential oil in meditative spaces, yoga studios, and more for a sense of relaxation and peace that is rarely found.

Tension is no match for neroli or petitgrain. If you need a middle note tension tamer, petitgrain is the divine conqueror desired. A neroli-based bath oil is particularly suited to tension-relieving baths. A note of caution: bath oils can cause unsafe conditions if they are not handled properly; lay down a nonstick mat or decals in the tub before filling it with water and oil, and wash out the tub after your bath as soon as possible.

Tension Tamer Bath Oil

Add the desired amount of this blend to warm bathwater to soothe aching muscles.

- 3 drops neroli essential oil (*Citrus aurantium*) for antianxiety, sedative, tension reducing
- 3 drops clary sage essential oil (*Salvia sclarea*) for antianxiety, knowledge, harmony
- 3 drops sandalwood essential oil (*Santalum album*) for protection, harmony, calming

Add the three essential oils to an 8-ounce glass bottle and fill halfway with your carrier oil of choice. Cap and shake gently before adding desired amount to warm running water. Enjoy!

High Priestess Oil

Use this blend to feel queenly, divine, and in charge.

- 10 drops neroli essential oil (*Citrus aurantium*) for protection, releasing negative emotions, stress relief
- 1 drop cinnamon leaf essential oil (*Cinnamomum verum*) for power, luck, protection
- 10 drops frankincense essential oil (*Boswellia carteri*) for protection, blessing, balance
- 1 drop rose absolute (*Rosa damascene*) for inner growth, love, protection, stimulated awareness

Based on the oil the British monarchy uses to anoint a new ruler, this empowering blend will make every meeting and project the stage fit for a queen. (For a more kingly version, substitute oakmoss absolute for rose.)

Blend all oils in a glass bottle and add 2 drops synergy to a 10 ml roller bottle filled with carrier oil to anoint.

Self-Improvement

Use this blend while striving to be a better person.

20 drops neroli essential oil (*Citrus aurantium*) for protection, releasing negative emotions, shielding

8 drops benzoin essential oil (*Styrax tonkinensis*) for exorcism, bringing balance

1 drop rosemary essential oil (*Rosmarinus officinalis*) for character, confidence, transformation

This blend smells like a sweet dessert just begging to be devoured. That will make this oil all the more effective when change is desired. It is often a difficult road, carved out of the brush with a machete. An oil that is sweet, comforting, and gentle will help ensure that not only is it effective for the chosen change but it will also provide a smooth transition.

Blend all oils and diffuse 1 drop synergy per 100 ml water during times of trial and turmoil to ensure strength and luck.

Dilute 1 drop synergy in a 10 ml bottle to anoint the proper candle. Figure candles are ideal for personal change, as many changes start within the self—but figures are not required, nor are candles, as the magic lies within the practitioner, not the materials used. For personal transformation in an ongoing struggle, add a drop of synergy to an aroma locket to be worn daily. Refresh as needed. Each time the aroma is noted, take a second to offer thanks. Gratitude goes a long way in magic.

Lammas Leavening

Diffuse this synergy for observances of the first harvest.

15 drops neroli essential oil (*Citrus aurantium*) to sedate, release negative emotional attachments, shield, reduce impact of trauma, relieve stress

15 drops benzoin essential oil (*Styrax tonkinensi*) for inspiration, harmony, love, memory, peace, purification

1 drop cinnamon essential oil (*Cinnamomum verum*) for good luck, protection, lifted spirits

35 drops vanilla absolute (*Vanilla planifolia*) for mental powers, relaxation, peace

Lammas or Lughnasadh usually takes place during the first harvest, the grain harvest. Traditionally celebrated at sundown on the first of August, breads are prepared and a portion is left out as a thanks for a bountiful harvest. Diffuse this warm scent for increasing the peace, luck, and harmony of a home. Anoint a candle with this blend for rituals of gratitude any time of the year. Consider a weekly or monthly gratitude practice.

A Note on Vanilla Essential Oil

Look for vanilla absolute or vanilla CO2 for purity standards. This is an expensive oil, and as such it is often adulterated. True vanilla will not smell like the sugar cookie air freshener found in the candle store. It will smell more like an old library. When paper breaks down, it produces an aldehyde chemical called vanillin when the paper ages, so named for the scent of natural vanilla. When people say they love the smell of old books, they really are admiring the scent of vanilla.

Nutmeg

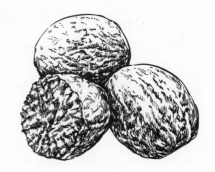

Scientific name: *Myristica fragrans*

Botanical family: Myristicaceae

Origin: Indonesia

Source of plant's oil: Fruit and seeds

Evaporation: Middle note

Scent description: Sharp, spicy, dark, warming

Scent impact: Banish fatigue

Magical Correspondences

Application: Diffuse, direct inhalation

Element: Fire

Day: Thursday

Magical uses: Money, luck, fidelity

Planet: Jupiter

Astrological sign: Sagittarius

Suggested crystal: Blue topaz—ruled by Sagittarius: speak your truth

Deities/spirits: Maman Brigitte, Vodou goddess of the dead; Brighid, Celtic goddess of inspiration and healing

Warnings

Do not use with children. Use sparingly, as it is a skin sensitizer.

HERBAL LORE

Nutmeg has been used far longer than recorded history. The earliest records of nutmeg's benefit state that nutmeg had already been used for hundreds of years in embalming practices in ancient Egypt by the time recipes and records were written down. During the Middle Ages, nutmeg was mixed with fatty ointment as a cure for diarrhea, nausea, muscle cramps, and other digestive issues.

As with all warming herbs, nutmeg is conflated with magic of love, sex, and fidelity.

USES

Place a drop of nutmeg essential oil in a water diffuser for magic invoking calm, rational thinking.

To banish harmful dreams and stimulate beneficial dream states, diffuse a drop of nutmeg essential oil in the bedroom up to thirty minutes before retiring for the evening. (Having a diffuser with an automatic shutoff is helpful.)

To bring good luck, anoint the bottoms of your shoes for the day with a drop of nutmeg essential oil diluted in a 10 ml roller bottle filled with the carrier oil of your choice. Using the roller bottle to draw a sigil for the form the luck takes is an extra step (pun intended) toward the luck of the day. Dollar symbols, stars, and coins are all appropriate signs. Walk with confidence throughout the day, knowing every step leaves its mark, working prosperity.

Nutmeg carries the loving energies of fidelity. If loyalty is needed in friendship, in marriage, or in business, inscribe a gold, orange, or yellow (success) candle with the word "fidelity" and anoint it with diluted nutmeg essential oil. Burn the candle on a Sunday (success).

Prosperity is the result of warming feelings exciting the needs of anyone involved. To invite prosperity, carve a green (money) or brown (stability) candle with the asset or dollar amount needed and anoint with diluted nutmeg essential oil. Burn the candle on a Sunday (success).

Needing physical or emotional strength? Turn to nutmeg for the muscles to handle anything coming down the pike. Diffuse a drop of nutmeg essential oil while making a list of ways to empower the required strength.

No matter how well we treat our bodies, time passes. For magic useful in averting arthritis and pain, anoint a brown candle (stability) and burn on a Thursday (protected growth).

To expand awareness past the boundaries of the physical form, diffuse nutmeg essential oil while meditating.

Divination and meditation benefit from the use of nutmeg. Nutmeg was burned in temples as a divinatory incense for the priests or priestesses to interpret. In the modern era, diffusing a drop of nutmeg essential oil and watching the trail of water vapor leaving the diffuser is an easier method, and without the potential hazards of smoke affecting the breathing of asthmatic patients or those with other breathing difficulties. (See the section on divination at the end of the book for more on scrying.)

Need to get down to business? Diffusing nutmeg can help increase focus and fuel creativity to make sure deadlines are reached and new ideas are always flowing.

Nutmeg is a potent ally for work involving hex breaking. If a hex is suspected, diffuse nutmeg oil in the home or make this simple nutmeg room spray: Place 1 teaspoon table salt in a glass bowl and add roughly 30 drops of nutmeg essential oil. Stir well. Pour the salt into a spray bottle and fill with enough water, sufficiently warm, to dissolve the salt. Give it a good shake before spraying.

Good health is within reach. To guard your family against illness (the start of flu season or the school year is an opportune time), take a copy of a family photo and around the border write "Health-HealthHealth" until your family is completely encircled. Using nutmeg anointing oil in a roller bottle, draw a circle around your family and outside of the handwritten health border. Once a week anoint the photo with a drop of nutmeg oil to keep the power of the enchantment going.

The same procedure can be used to protect the home, whether you're going away on vacation or conspiring against everyday worries of severe weather, vandalism, or robbery. The entire family can be pictured in front of the home, or not. Both are acceptable.

When justice is called upon, nutmeg answers. If a just judge is needed, anoint a blue candle (balance) with nutmeg oil and burn on a Thursday (protected growth). To justly banish a bogus lawsuit, anoint a black candle (banishing) with diluted nutmeg oil and burn on a Saturday (endings). Burn during the waning or new moons for added benefit.

To banish negative memories and remember happier times, diffuse nutmeg essential oil. Picture negative memories as pieces of paper being balled up in a fist and thrown into a black hole. See their impact diminishing with each paper thrown in.

Trance states and visions are easier to attain with movement and scent enhancers. To benefit a visionary practice, try adding walking, dancing, or movement while listening to drumming and diffusing nutmeg essential oil in a water diffuser.

Into the Dreaming

Use when encouraging prophetic or meaningful dreams.

>   5 drops nutmeg (*Myristica fragrans*) for dreaming, good luck, strength, clairvoyance

>   3 drops cedarwood (*Cedrus atlantica*) for clairvoyance, consecration, divination, success

>   15 drops lemon (*Citrus limon*) for calming clarity, blessings, ability

Need to understand how a situation developed? Working to see where choices will lead a year from now? Diffuse 1 drop of this synergy in 100 ml water up to thirty minutes before bed to encourage dreams of a far-seeing or divinatory purpose. For added benefit, dilute a drop in a 2 ml bottle of carrier before anointing a yellow candle (success) on a Sunday (success) before attempting journeywork through dreams.

Oakmoss

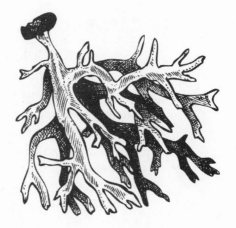

Scientific name: *Evernia furfuracea*

Botanical family: Parmeliaceae

Origin: Morocco

Source of plant's oil: Solvent extracted from lichen (tree moss)

Evaporation: Base note

Scent description: Warm, woody, leather, violet

Scent impact: Soothing, grounding

Magical Correspondences

Application: Diffuse, topical with low dilution

Element: Earth

Day: Friday

Magical uses: Divination, exorcism, grounding

Planet: Venus

Astrological sign: Taurus

Suggested crystal: Zoisite—ruled by Gemini: chase away lethargy

Deity/spirit: Pazuzu, apotropaion god of exorcism

Warnings

Skin sensitizer. Can irritate mucosal linings. Toxic in large doses. Do not use above 1 to 2 percent dilution. Should not be used by those with seizure disorders or a history of panic attacks.

HERBAL LORE

Oakmoss is a lichen that attaches itself to oak and other rough-barked trees, and is used as a fixative in potpourri. This moss-like fungi soaks up oils well and is decorative enough for potpourri. This small gray-green member of the kingdom of fungi yields a dark green, thick absolute. Since it is used as a fixative in perfume, the staying power can also be used in magic. Folk magic practitioners stuff poppets with oakmoss to make their magic have a longer-lasting effect. You can get this by placing a drop of oakmoss absolute on a cotton ball and adding it to stuffing when making a poppet.

Oakmoss Absolute

"Absolute" is the designation for oils that are derived from solvent extraction for materials that are too delicate for steam distillation. (For more information, see Extracting Essential Oils on page 16 and Appendix D: Botanical Magic Resources.) Due to the viscous nature of oakmoss absolute, a water bath may be necessary. Place the unopened bottle in a cup of warm water for a few minutes prior to use. Not only will this allow the bottle to open more easily, but it will make the absolute less viscous and easier to work with. Drops will be difficult to count, because this oil is really thick. Add oakmoss last and shake well to incorporate.

USES

For clairvoyant experiences, blend oakmoss absolute with a meditative essential oil or two, such as neroli or ylang-ylang, and diffuse the synergy while searching the inner self for answers. If attempting to diffuse outside of a synergy, proceed with caution; the viscous nature of this oil may gum up small electrical diffusers. An older style oil burner that works on a candle may be more beneficial; just use fire safety protocols. This method can also be used for contacting other planes and divination of many kinds.

A potent tool for hex breaking and exorcism, dried oakmoss can be added to a poppet for direct work. The absolute blends well to make an exorcism oil that packs a punch (see Hex-Shattering Oil on page 105).

Immensely grounding and centering, this fungi can root people in the here and now as well as aid in contacting spirits of the forest and individual trees. To gain more grounding, diffuse a drop of oakmoss absolute in water with an oil burner, or create a poppet to represent yourself. Once it is named, anoint the feet of the doll with diluted oakmoss oil. Keep this doll safe, and make sure to give it a date when it becomes inactive and is no longer an extension of you.

Oakmoss can yield long-term results when used for business, manifesting, and prosperity work, specifically for money and good luck. Since oakmoss is a fixative, it is not a resource that is quickly burned out. Slow and steady is the motto here. Add oakmoss to prosperity oils for a lasting effect.

My Mistress's Eyes

Use to divine the face of future lovers or in magic to draw new love.

4 drops oakmoss absolute (*Evernia furfuracea*) for divination, luck, manifestation

30 drops amber essential oil (*Pinus succinifera*) for attraction, happiness, love, soul mates

20 drops petitgrain essential oil (*Citrus aurantium*) for joy, purification, transformation

Diffuse 1 drop synergy in 100 ml water a half hour before bed to dream of the next lover to grace your boudoir. Dilute 1 drop synergy in 2 ml carrier oil to anoint a candle and ask the universe to bring you the next love on the way. Remember, oakmoss absolute is thick and sticky, so shake the bottle hard to incorporate the absolute before diffusing or diluting.

Ex-Breaking Banishing Oil

Old lover turning up like a bad penny?

- 2 drops oakmoss absolute (*Evernia furfuracea*) for exorcism, luck
- 1 drop clove essential oil (*Syzygium aromaticum*) for hex breaking, dispelling negativity, protection
- 15 drops frankincense essential oil (*Boswellia carteri*) for banishing, purification
- 1 drop tangerine essential oil (*Citrus reticulate*) for defense

Mix all oils and dilute 1 drop synergy in a 2 ml bottle and fill with carrier oil of choice. Anoint an orange candle with the oil, and burn it on a Saturday to make sure your ex does not return.

Orange (Sweet)

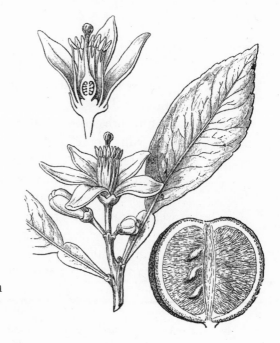

Scientific name: *Citrus sinensis*

Botanical family: Rutaceae

Origin: China, South America, Italy

Source of plant's oil: Peels

Evaporation: Top note

Scent description: Sweet, bright, citrus, caramel

Scent impact: Relax, combat depression

Magical Correspondences

Application: Diffuse, direct inhalation, topically with care

Element: Fire

Day: Sunday

Magical uses: Joy, prosperity, attraction, beauty, sensuality

Planet: Sun

Astrological sign: Leo

Suggested crystal: Rhondite—ruled by Taurus: balancing male and female energies

Deity/spirit: Adrestia, Greek goddess of divine balance

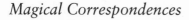

Warnings

Sweet orange is sensitizing; do not use in dilutions of over 1 percent (1 drop per 5 ml carrier oil) for skin safety. In large doses its aroma can cause tiredness and lethargy.

HERBAL LORE

Oranges (and most natural citrus plants) originated in China. Sweet orange did not make its way to its current home in South Africa until the fifteenth century, when trade routes brought these divinely associated fruits to the land.

Sweet orange essential oil, derived from cold pressing the peel, is ideal for any magical work involving purification due to its acidic properties. The fiery and solar associations burn away impurities as well as traits and situations that no longer benefit us.

The doctrine of signatures dating from the time of Paracelsus, in the early 1500s, tells us that every plant was autographed by God with a road map for use. Carrots contain an eye, so are useful for vision. Yellow is the color of bile, so yellow flowers can benefit the liver. The same can be said for magic. Golden-colored plants, oils, and flowers can be utilized for prosperity and success. If a plant is capable of protecting itself with spines or thorns (like roses or brambles) or a thick outer skin (like oranges), then it is well suited for protection magic.

As mentioned with neroli, citrus has been associated with goddess of home and hearth and as such makes an excellent partner for beauty as well.

USES

Place a drop of sweet orange oil in an aroma locket to entice love and attraction. A gentle yet effective love spell involves using diluted sweet orange oil to anoint a candle. Light it while creating a list of traits in an ideal partner. Include things that are important, but do not make the list so specific that it makes the spell ineffective.

Looking to engage the inner Eros or Aphrodite? Sweet orange is an oil of eroticism and sensuality. Recognizing the sensuous nature of the self is separate from seeing the beauty in the self. When it is time to turn the lights down, diffuse a drop of sweet orange oil to remember where those feelings originate.

Orange is also associated with beauty. Dilute 1 drop sweet orange essential oil in a 10 ml roller bottle and apply behind the ears. This will remind you of your inherent beauty inside and out.

In need of good luck? Turn to sweet orange. The doctrine of signatures reminds us that items of the natural world that are gold can attract good luck as well as prosperity. To turn the tide of luck in a favorable direction, anoint an orange candle with diluted sweet orange oil. Using a ballpoint pen, carve a word or symbol describing the luck needed (e.g., getting a contract, getting pregnant, kicking a run of bad luck) into the candle. Burn the candle on a Sunday.

Diffuse a drop of sweet orange essential oil in 100 ml water before attempting to make a baby. A stress-relieving scent plus the magic of fertility equals a winning combination. Anoint a candle with diluted sweet orange oil to further increase fertility.

To spark happiness, engage the scent of orange oil. Peel and eat an orange, visualizing the sweetness of life. Diffuse sweet orange essential oil in spaces frequented, as well as emotionally charged spaces to lighten the mood (talk therapy offices, medical offices, and ecclesiastical spaces).

To restore harmony, reach for sweet orange oil. Diffuse one drop of sweet orange essential oil in 100 ml water where all parties will be present.

The stimulating effect of sweet orange oil can also be used to spur action and gain momentum. Whether there is a project that needs to get done by a deadline, or it is simply difficult to get off the ground, reach for the action of sweet orange oil. A gentle direct inhalation over the bottle once an hour will help with an energy boost. Diffuse a drop of sweet orange in a well-ventilated space (let us not make the entire group fall asleep) during planning meetings and while assigning duties for a project. Not only will it help keep everyone engaged, but every time they smell oranges after that they will remember the job assigned. So if one member of the group starts shirking duties or falling behind, simply offer them a cup of orange tea or a slice of an orange to remind them of their commitments.

If used in slightly higher doses, orange can cause deep sleep. The bonus portion of that action is that the intersection of antianxiety, depression lifting, and calming effects all work together to create beneficial dreams without the emotional turmoil of night terrors. Adding 3 or 4 drops of sweet orange oil to a small room diffuser a half hour before bed will bring sweet dreams.

Flexibility and adaptability are the hallmarks of a valuable employee and a respected romantic partner. When it comes time to remember how to be flexible, diffuse sweet orange oil while making a list of ways to be adaptable in day-to-day life while still maintaining healthy boundaries. Remember, one cannot serve from an empty vessel; self-care is important as well.

Wishing to feel ambitious? Let the light of the sunshine in. Sweet orange oil can lend those energies out easily. Peel and eat an orange, embracing the scent of the orange peel with each piece of peel removed. Visualize yourself setting achievable goals and accomplishing them. Alternately, diffuse sweet orange oil while meditating on the nature of ambition.

Aura feeling a bit murky and muddy? Add a drop or two of sweet orange essential oil to 1 tablespoon salt and stir well. Draw a warm bath and sprinkle the salt in the bath. Soak in the purifying waters for as long as desired and step out of the bath feeling refreshed and whole.

Authority is 10 percent bestowed and 90 percent assumed. If the authority has been accorded but the confidence is not there to back it up, it can result in a vote of no confidence. Step up and claim that crown with sweet orange oil. An aroma necklace will come in handy in this situation, as every time the orange scent registers in your brain you can stop, square those shoulders, adjust the crown of your head, and remember whom others are dealing with. The confidence and self-worth boost bestowed by sweet orange can also help make it clear who is boss. Reclaim the power.

The solar success of sweet orange makes it an ideal help for court cases. If you find yourself going to court, make a copy of the first page of the official papers. Turn it over and write the name of the respondent six times. Turn the paper 90 degrees and write your name on top of theirs six times. Anoint with sweet orange anointing oil and place under an orange candle. Burn the candle on a Tuesday for confidence and success. Orange is built for overcoming problems.

In matters of the creative spirit, diffuse sweet orange essential oil in creation spaces—art studios, writing offices, even yoga studios.

Sweet orange oil is uplifting and supports the weight of depression. Medications may still be required, and talk therapy is beneficial, but allow the bolstering support of a calming antianxiety oil like sweet orange to help out.

Divination with sweet orange is a snap. Water scrying, by placing a drop of sweet orange oil in a darkly colored bowl, can act as a focus for the work. Just softly focus your eyes as though you were looking at a Magic Eye picture, and breathe slowly and deeply. Allow images to form in your mind. Another method is to incorporate air by watching the water and sweet orange oil mist coming out of a water diffuser and allowing the mind to wander.

Sweet orange oil is associated with release and healing. However, it is not the quiet, soothing healing that lavender provides. Sweet orange is a solar oil; associated with fire, it will act quickly and powerfully to banish illness. Shred the threads of that illness by diffusing the oil in a sickroom or anointing a candle with diluted sweet orange with the target of the healing's name written on it.

Prosperity Abounds Spell

To ask for increased prosperity, or material objects, gather a healthy plant, a pot to grow it in, and paper to write on. Detail the need, whether it's a steady income or a home large enough for the family. Anoint the paper with sweet orange essential oil and place it in the bottom of the new pot. Scoop a few handfuls of soil into the pot and place the plant into the pot. Continue to place handfuls of earth into the pot until it is filled properly and water it. As the plant grows, so will the prosperity.

Harmony Spell

Do a Google image search for the Ten of Pentacles tarot card and print it on regular paper. Cut out the image, and on the back of the paper write about the situation at hand—how it came to be out of balance and what can happen to restore harmony. Place 1 drop of sweet orange oil on each corner of the tarot card photo and place it under a candle. Burn the candle on a Monday (for comfort and emotional security).

Lasting Love

Use this oil when love is new and sweet to ground it in the long term.

10 drops sweet orange essential oil (*Citrus sinensis*) for harmony, love, luck, beauty, sensuality

5 drops Persian lime essential oil (*Citrus latifolia*) for friendship, fidelity

5 drops oakmoss absolute (*Evernia furfuracea*) for grounding, manifestation

Blend oils in a 2 ml glass bottle. Repeat to fill, if desired. Diffuse 1 drop synergy per 100 ml water during quiet nights in to encourage bonding and sharing.

Alternatively, add 1 to 2 drops synergy to a 10 ml roller bottle and fill with carrier oil to make an anointing oil.

Raining Sunshine

Increase prosperity and lift spirits with this blend.

10 drops sweet orange essential oil (*Citrus sinensis*) for good luck, prosperity, material objects

4 drops bergamot essential oil (*Citrus bergamia*) for attraction, money, prosperity, strength

5 drops fennel essential oil (*Foeniculum vulgare*) for protection, truth

5 drops patchouli essential oil (*Pogostemon cablin*) to increase the power of spells, protection

Worrying about money is a common event, but worrying is detrimental. Stress and fatigue are rampant and can lead to feelings of helplessness. Next time you're paying bills, boost your mood and make way for prosperity with this oil.

Mix all oils in a 2 ml bottle. Either diffuse 1 drop synergy per 100 ml water, or fill the bottle with carrier oil and use it for anointing candles, charms, talismans, and copies of financial planning documents.

Choral Bells

Use this uplifting oil to remind yourself of beauty and joy.

10 drops sweet orange essential oil (*Citrus sinensis*) for beauty, strength, happiness

5 drops clary sage essential oil (*Salvia sclarea*) for retention, harmony

6 drops lavender essential oil (*Lavandula angustifolia*) for balance, peace

5 drops tangerine essential oil (*Citrus reticulate*) for antidepressant, defense

Bells have been used throughout history to invoke glad tidings and joy and clear the air of negativity. Feel the chorus of gods, angels, faeries, and other beings uplifting and supporting during stressful times with this blend.

Mix all oils together and diffuse 1 drop synergy per 100 ml water during difficult times to be reminded of joy.

Patchouli

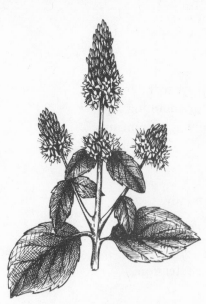

Scientific name: *Pogostemon cablin*

Botanical family: Lamiaceae

Origin: India

Source of plant's oil: Fermented leaves

Evaporation: Base note

Scent description: Earthy, warm, loamy

Scent impact: Grounding, gain clarity of thought

Magical Correspondences

Application: Diffuse, direct inhalation, topical with dilution

Element: Earth

Day: Saturday

Magical uses: Aphrodisiac, prosperity, boosting magical efficacy

Planets: Saturn, Pluto

Astrological signs: Scorpio, Capricorn

Suggested crystal: Unakite—ruled by Scorpio: grounding and balance

Deity/spirit: Demeter, Greek goddess of grains (associated with grounding)

Warnings

Appetite suppressant—avoid if you are ill or have an eating disorder.

HERBAL LORE

The scent of patchouli is a historic one, reaching back hundreds of years before the psychedelic era it's most commonly associated with. When textiles were shipped from India to England, the lush fabrics were layered with patchouli leaves to protect them from insects during the long months at sea. Patchouli developed an association with luxury, money, and beauty as a result. The fact that patchouli is antimicrobial and therefore kept the material from molding or rotting was also a factor that leads to associations with protection.

Patchouli is associated with another export of India: Indian ink. Patchouli and camphor are the principal materials that give Indian ink its signature scent. This makes traditional Indian ink perfect for writing out money spells.

USES

Patchouli can be used to stem the tide of rising aggression. Diffuse one drop of patchouli oil in a space occupied by the aggressor. Alternatively, place 1 drop patchouli essential oil in a 2 ml bottle and fill with the carrier oil of your choice. Whisper the name of the aggressor to a candle and anoint it with diluted patchouli oil. Burn the candle on a Tuesday if possible for added effect.

Patchouli is an herb of attraction. From lovers to customers, patchouli brings the desired outcome. Diffuse patchouli while using a guided meditation to direct the focus of the outcome. See a business full of customers, see a new love entering the picture, and more. With patchouli's associations of growth it is especially beneficial for attracting customers, clients, and business. Patchouli is also used for luck, manifestation, and prosperity of all kinds.

Speaking of attraction, the grounding actions of this earthy herb drop the awareness to the lower chakras, where sexual desire originates. To encourage sexual desires, diffuse a drop or two of patchouli essential oil in a room thirty minutes to an hour before hoping to entice a lover. Note: this in no way impedes the free will of another—the aphrodisiac qualities of patchouli merely signal interest to the potential lover. Affirmative consent, first and foremost. Yes means yes.

The grounding effects of patchouli can also be applied in other ways. Patchouli is adept at grounding unacceptable behavior and has long been used in magic to rid oneself of bad habits and addictions. While magic is no substitute for licensed treatment programs, magic can give strength and support to those afflicted. If you're trying to face a bad habit or addiction, choose a candle that represents the strength of being free of the habit. For example, try peach (peace) for nail biting or addiction, and brown (stability) for smoking, drinking, or using drugs. Do not choose a candle to represent the addiction (e.g., dice for gambling addicts), as this can reinforce negative behavior. Dilute 1 drop of patchouli essential oil in a 2 ml bottle of the carrier oil of choice. Anoint the candle representing newfound strength and burn it on a Sunday for strength, the full moon for power, or a Tuesday for victory.

If a loved one is facing a long recovery (broken bones, surgery, or illness) use patchouli to give them strength. Diffuse during visits to keep their spirits up. Burn a candle anointed with diluted patchouli oil to ask healing gods to smile upon them. Remember to keep visits short, as they may tire easily. And do not expect them to be the best host or have a spotless home if they are dealing with a serious illness, autoimmune disease, or broken bones. Instead of judging, offer to do the dishes, or bring a meal along for the ride so that they do not feel compelled to feed or care for guests.

Patchouli can help both aims because of its earthy scent. It is a reminder that we live in the here and now, and that time travel (worrying about the future or living in the past) is the root of all suffering. Take slow, deep breaths while a drop of patchouli oil is diffused in the room and be in the moment. Thoughts will pop up. Just let them pass on by.

Learning to quiet those inner voices will come in handy. Learning to be still and quiet is the first step to working with the intuition we all possess. When attempting to expand one's clairvoyance (clear seeing) or clairaudience (clear hearing), contact other planes of existence, or practice divination of any kind, patchouli is a powerful oil to reach for. Diffuse patchouli oil while divining to stretch those wings and grow as an intuitive.

The grounding properties of patchouli are also beneficial for exorcism, hex breaking, and banishing, making this oil ideal for consecration and purification rituals. Nature abhors a vacuum, so when one energy is banished it makes room for the opposite end of the spectrum to flow in. Anoint sacred tools with a dot of diluted patchouli oil to encourage sacred energy. (Beware the diluted oil can damage the finish on wood. Use caution. Do a patch test if needed.) Diffuse patchouli oil to consecrate ritual space in place of incense for people with asthma.

Patchouli is a commanding herb. It not only breaks jinxes, hexes, and curses but can also act to bring other things into being. Overly amorous suitor? Command them to leave you alone by writing "back

Grounding and Centering

Grounding and centering are discussed often in magical and energy-rich circles. Grounding is connecting with the earth to rid the body of excess energy, or to draw additional energy from the earth to sustain proper levels of functionality. Centering is the practice of joining all of the disparate forms of energy throughout the body in the very center of the being. Stretch those visualization techniques by seeing threads of scattered energy in the body smoothing and coming together in the center of the body, and then connecting with the earth. A gentle give and take, the earth can take when you have too much, and give if you have a need.

off, (name)!" on a piece of paper dressed with patchouli oil. Bury it off of your property to ground their affections.

One drop of patchouli oil in a 2 ml bottle filled with carrier oil will act as a powerful protective aid, psychically. Patchouli is also used for scar repair and other beneficial skin uses, so it should not bother skin as long as it is properly diluted.

If worries are plaguing you day and night, not only is patchouli an antidepressant and antianxiety source, but the magical properties encouraging peace of mind are battle tested. Find a candle of a soothing color and anoint it after writing "peace" on it with a pen. Light the candle while diffusing patchouli oil and practicing intentional breath work.

Fair treatment is another hallmark of patchouli. To be assigned a fair judge in a court case, inscribe "Fair Judge" on a candle and anoint with diluted patchouli oil. Burn the candle on a Tuesday (for victory) during the waxing moon. The first page (the complaint) of a set of court documents can be copied and anointed with patchouli for a fair judge, and as an oil of defense, it can only help the case. If this route is taken, place the copy underneath the fireproof container that the candle is burning safely inside of. (For more court magic, see page 175 in the Jasmine section.)

Patchouli oil and the dried herb are both utilized to increase the power of spells. Add a leaf to mojo bags or other charms to increase the power of spells. In the case of candle magic, add a pinch of patchouli herb inside the base of a taper candleholder where it can add its own energy without being a fire hazard. Some attempt to anoint candles and then roll them in ground or dried herbs. These herbs are still flammable and can pose a risk of fire. Alternately, if using tea lights, pull the candle out of the small tin they are shipped in, place a small pinch inside the cup, and replace the candle. The energy of the patchouli will still be there, and it will be covered in melting wax as it melts. This means that it is not until the candle is nearly burned out that the herbs can potentially burn, and by then it is perfectly acceptable to blow out the candle and dispose of the remains.

Love Drawing Bath

Patchouli's relationship with love, sex, lust, fertility, and passion is well documented. In folk magic practices around the world patchouli is added to love drawing baths. Fill a muslin tea bag with dried patchouli and a tablespoon of the salt of choice (for purifying) and tie closed. Toss into a running bath of warm water and soak up the loving vibrations. Patchouli also helps to increase libido, so feel free to share this bath with a lover whose libido has taken a dip.

Remembrance Oil

Halloween or Samhain (pronounced SOW-en) is the time of the year most commonly associated with remembering the dead, but it is not the only time our loved ones can cross the veil to visit with us and watch over our lives. To remember deceased loved ones, choose a candle in their favorite color and inscribe it with their name or a nickname. Anoint the candle with diluted patchouli oil and set it up in a place of honor in the home with a photo, if possible. Burn the candle anytime that connection is desired, as well as at birthdays, anniversaries, and Halloween.

Unleash all that bottled up creativity. All that grounding and love focus the intent by releasing imagination. Diffuse a drop or two of patchouli essential oil in creative spaces, art studios, or offices—especially for projects that are a labor of love.

The antianxiety and antidepressant properties of this oil also make it an exemplary tool for harmony, balance, and happiness. Troubles are put away, making room for the warmth and contentment of true happiness. Wear a drop of patchouli essential oil in an aroma locket for a reminder that happiness is a gift from the universe and harmony is possible. Diffuse patchouli oil in high-traffic areas to reestablish a happy home.

All that grounding has to be good for something besides smelling incredibly earthy and warm. Along with banishing evil, patchouli can banish the evils of illness. For magic involving banishing illnesses, colds, or the flu, diffuse patchouli essential oil in the home in common areas. Dilute 1 drop of patchouli essential oil in 10 ml carrier oil and anoint doorknobs inside and out, sink knobs, and the backs of mirrors in the home. Run the garbage disposal with the hottest water out of the tap and add a drop or two down the disposal while you're at it. Patchouli is not just antimicrobial; it is also antibacterial.

Attempting to master a new skill? Patchouli's earthly connections make it a natural for increasing memory and therefore mastering a new skill or ability. To improve memory and mastery, diffuse patchouli essential oil while learning and practicing a new skill. If diffusing will not work in the present environment, add a drop to an aroma locket and wear it under your clothes while working. The warmth from your body will diffuse the aroma just enough for benefit, without smelling like a hippie.

Bodily Acceptance Working

Patchouli has been used to soften scar tissue and help with scar revision and healing. Instead of looking at this plant as changing us, let us embrace it as healing acceptance.

Dilute 1 drop of patchouli essential oil in a 10 ml roller bottle of the carrier oil of choice. (Remember to patch test twenty-four hours beforehand on a small spot of slightly more sensitive skin, such as the inside of the wrist or elbow.)

With or without a mirror, this working is magical and transformative. Look at your body as a whole. Are there places that make you cringe? If so, these are the places that need the most love. Use the roller bottle to draw hearts, words of acceptance, and other symbols on lines, wrinkles, scars, excess skin or fat, and anything else that makes you feel less than amazing. Because you are amazing. Say it out loud. Your body has been through a lot, and it is still kicking. Once any piece that is upsetting is drawn on, cap the roller bottle and massage all the oil into the skin while telling yourself things you love about your body. Once you're finished, lounge around in a robe, pamper yourself, and relax.

Payment Due

Has a friend borrowed money and not yet repaid you? Is it starting to impact the friendship?

- 15 drops patchouli essential oil (*Pogostemon cablin*) for commanding, money, power

- 26 drops lime essential oil (*Citrus latifolia*) for friendship, strength

- 3 drops rosemary essential oil (*Rosmarinus officinalis*) for confidence, character, courage

Mix all oils and diffuse 1 drop synergy per 100 ml water before your friend comes over, or once they have arrived. Alternately, place 1 drop synergy in a 2 ml bottle and fill with a carrier oil of choice. Anoint a candle with this oil to ask for the swift return of funds. Burn the candle on a Wednesday for communication or Thursday for money during the waxing moon.

Grounding Anxiety

Simply being able to breathe can feel like magic. Use this blend when you need to take a moment to breathe.

- 4 drops patchouli essential oil (*Pogostemon cablin*) for balance, centering, grounding, harmony

- 3 drops clary sage essential oil (*Salvia sclarea*) for balance, harmony, wisdom, clarity

- 5 drops tangerine essential oil (*Citrus reticulata*) for calming, antidepressant, protection

Place oils in a 1-ounce glass or number 1 plastic bottle and gently stir. Fill the bottle with the carrier oil of choice, cap, and shake. Use this oil to anoint the heart chakra when anxiety feels overwhelming. Make a second batch in a 2 ml bottle without the carrier oil to diffuse in spaces frequently attended, such as your living room, bedroom (for a great night's sleep), and office (if allowed).

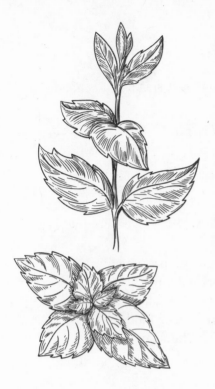

Peppermint

Scientific name: *Mentha piperita*

Botanical family: Lamiaceae

Origin: North America

Source of plant's oil: Leaves

Evaporation: Top note

Scent description: Cool, herbal, refreshing

Scent impact: Awaken the mind

Magical Correspondences

Application: Diffuse, dilute, topical application

Element: Air

Day: Wednesday

Magical uses: Psychic development, purification, release, good luck

Planet: Mercury

Astrological sign: Gemini

Suggested crystal: Topaz—ruled by Sagittarius: empowerment and successful endeavors

Deity/spirit: Zeus, father of the Greek gods

Warnings

Do not use on or around children under five years of age. Can result in fatal breathing lapses and suffocation. Bathing with peppermint essential oil is not recommended, and do not use in dilutions higher than 1 percent, as burns and irritation can occur. Inhalation of large doses can lead to dizziness, confusion, nausea, double vision, muscle weakness, and other symptoms.

Herbal Lore

Peppermint is one of the herbs reputed to have been a part of the Four Thieves Vinegar of Marseilles. (See Clove for a recipe.) The magical and medicinal uses of peppermint have long revolved around the purification of the mint family. Doctors would tell patients to rub fresh leaves on their heads to relieve headaches, and modern headache essential oil rollers contain peppermint and lavender synergies.

The older name of the mint family Labiatae refers to the flower shape resembling the shape of female genetalia and is therefore associated with love magic, like the members of the mint family such as basil, hyssop, lavender, marjoram, oregano, peppermint, rosemary, sage, savory, and thyme.

Uses

Hoping to gain an intellectual advantage at work? Reach for a bottle of peppermint essential oil. The mercurial, airy nature of peppermint connects it with intellectual stimulation and the ability to think on your feet. It stimulates alertness and is associated with change, so it will be difficult to throw you a curve ball. Diffuse peppermint essential oil at your desk for alertness, clear thinking, and rational discourse. Peppermint also banishes mental fatigue and laziness.

Ready to make the leap into action but feeling hampered by indecision? The mental acuity of peppermint paired with its stimulating action will be just the kick in the pants you need. Diffuse peppermint essential oil while making a list of projects to be completed and their desired deadlines. Anoint the paper with diluted peppermint oil (1 drop essential oil in a 10 ml roller bottle filled with carrier oil) and place it in a prominent place. Every time you see or smell the paper, go over the list and determine what can and should be being accomplished. Include ways to meet goals (including limiting exposure to social media, games, or time wasters).

Peppermint is the scent of awakening, both mentally and psychically. A scent associated with divination and mental prowess, use peppermint to open the hidden realms of the mind. Diffuse peppermint essential oil while practicing intentional breathing and test the limits of physical and psychic awareness. Peppermint expands perception outside of the physical realm.

Though life can sometimes feel like a competition in plate spinning, peppermint can help not only restore balance within the body between physical and mental stressors but also find balance within ourselves so that we may no longer need to rely on peppermint to do the work for us. When life seems overwhelming, diffuse peppermint and make a list of all the things that are under control and proceeding cleanly.

The sharp threads of peppermint make it an exemplary oil for banishing work. It can banish everything from negativity to indecision and sleeplessness. If banishing negativity, diffuse peppermint oil throughout affected areas. When banishing indecision, gently inhale directly over the bottle while making a list of pros and cons for the decision needed. If banishing sleeplessness, diffuse peppermint oil in the bedroom thirty minutes before retiring for bed, or place a drop or two on a tissue and place inside your pillowcase. Peppermint also creates sweet and beneficial dreams.

Embrace change with the help of peppermint. If life seems to be changing more and more rapidly and things are getting out of control, anoint a candle with diluted peppermint oil (1 drop essential oil in a 10 ml roller bottle filled with the carrier oil of your choice) and ask the universe to smooth things to a more manageable level.

Creative endeavors pair well with peppermint. It empowers creative thought and opens the gates to brainstorming new projects, establishing beneficial habits for creative expression and more. Diffuse peppermint in creative spaces, art studios, and writer's offices.

Doing magic to banish depression? Reach for a bottle of peppermint essential oil. Not only is peppermint an antidepressant, but it can also help banish the lethargy and mentality that often accompany depression. Diffuse peppermint oil to remember that though things may be difficult at the moment, they are temporary. Useful in conjunction with talk therapy and other interventions.

Bad habits are no match for peppermint. Make a list of the ways a bad habit is impacting your day-to-day life (e.g., expenses, time, alienating family, etc.). Anoint the list and a candle with diluted peppermint oil and burn the candle on a Tuesday for victory or a Wednesday for communication, or on a full moon.

Peppermint is used frequently in purification magic because it is high in menthol, eucalyptol, and other camphoraceous chemicals. It is a decongestant and expectorant. It comes as no surprise that these traits align peppermint with healing magic for colds, the flu, and other physical ailments. Diffuse peppermint in the sickroom of loved ones to banish the illness.

Try some poppet magic: Draw a gingerbread figure to act as a paper doll for healing work. Cut out the shape and name it after the sick child or family member. Apply diluted peppermint to the healing paper doll in the proper places (e.g., the forehead for fever, the nose for a sinus infection, etc.). Make sure to give the paper doll a date on the back when it will no longer be attached to the loved one. (For a simple cold, a week should be sufficient.) After the doll's date has passed and it is no longer connected to the loved one, burn it to ash so it cannot be used again. Peppermint is also an analgesic, so magic for pain relief is also appropriate.

Someone getting too comfortable on the couch, avoiding life in favor of video games, social media, or other time sucks? To get someone to engage with life again, write their name on a candle and anoint it with diluted peppermint oil. Burn the candle when the moon is waxing.

Love, lust, and passionate associations are some of the reasons why peppermint is sometimes thought of a Venusian herb. While it is still associated with Mercury, both connotations make it ideal for communicating with romantic partners. When discussing the emotional and physical needs of a relationship, relationship agreements, and communication styles, diffuse peppermint oil.

Power is just a drop away with peppermint. To empower charms, bags, talismans, and more, anoint with diluted peppermint oil. Bags may need a drop of peppermint every week or two to keep the energy flowing.

Need cooler heads to prevail after an argument? Diffuse peppermint to help restore clear thinking, remain coolheaded, and encourage loving consideration.

Peppermint is relaxing, and when paired with essential oils like lavender (*Lavandula angustifolia*) it is often suggested for headaches, allergies, sinusitis, and migraines. (With migraines, proceed gently, as some scents can trigger nausea. Peppermint should help with the nausea, but scents that are too strong can cause a gag reflex.) Magically, diffusing small amounts of peppermint essential oil can lend itself to banishing the punishing pains of headaches of many kinds.

Peppermint is also a scent of release. The airy relationships of peppermint and the associations of love make it a perfect friend to turn to when relationships end and the grief feels overwhelming. Curl up in a safe place with or without your favorite ice cream, and diffuse peppermint essential oil while making peace with the threads of the past. Peppermint is useful for renewal as well.

The expansion of self through perception, divination, and mental abilities is aided with the use of peppermint. Clairvoyance (clear seeing) is a skill that must be practiced in order to become proficient. Diffuse peppermint essential oil while training to sense auras. Partner exercises are beneficial here. Ask a friend to stand against a light-colored wall or door. Unfocus the eyes as though looking through the person. Eventually an outline will appear an inch to several feet away from their body. Once the outline is visible, attempt to discern colors around the person. This method can also be used to discern spirits. Visions are possible using peppermint essential oil for scrying as well. Meditate with peppermint tea to expand your consciousness.

Need help studying or otherwise focusing your attention? Intellectual strength, dedication, and persistence can be had with peppermint as an ally. Diffuse the essential oil at the table where study groups are meeting, and offer peppermint tea.

Peppermint is favorable in uncrossing work. Anything that smells sharp can cut through hexes, jinxes, and curses quickly. Peppermint has the added bonus of leaving positive vibrations in its wake and raising the energy of a space. Peppermint lends a warmth to a space that is unparalleled in such a cold scent. The magic of peppermint is transformation; embrace it.

Since peppermint is used in uncrossing work, it is a natural for consecration oils. It is uplifting both for the soul and the item being made sacred. Diluted essential oil will also scent wooden objects. (Test a small patch for color fastness first if the wood is finished.)

Peaceful Endings

Use this blend to make peace when relationships end.

- 1 drop peppermint essential oil (*Mentha piperita*) for healing, love, happiness

- 10 drops petitgrain essential oil (*Citrus aurantium*) for transformation, joy, banishing depression

- 20 drops sandalwood (*Santalum album*) for protection, harmony, honesty

Mix all oils in a 2 ml bottle. Diffuse synergy during comfort-seeking behaviors in the grief process. Dilute 1 drop synergy in 2 ml carrier oil to create an anointing oil for candle magic of a release, renewal, and emotional empowerment.

Petitgrain

See Neroli.

Rose

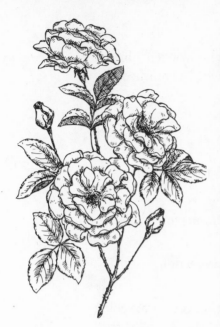

Scientific name: *Rosa damascena*

Botanical family: Rosaceae

Origin: Turkey

Source of plant's oil: Flowers

Evaporation: Middle note

Scent description: Heavy, warm, floral, hint of citrus

Scent impact: Achieve harmony, thoughts of love, sense of well-being

Magical Correspondences

Application: Topical, direct inhalation, diffusing

Element: Water

Day: Friday

Magical uses: Emotional uplifting, love, secrets, forgiveness

Planet: Venus

Astrological sign: Taurus

Suggested crystal: Diamond—ruled by Taurus: courage, strength, trust

Deity/spirit: Astarte, Greek goddess of sex, war, and fertility

Warnings

Avoid during pregnancy.

Herbal Lore

Associated with love, romance, and decadence, rose is one of the most recognizable scents in the world. But those slender, perfect, red rosebuds presented to lovers on Valentine's Day have little in common with the riotous, full, and beautiful pink buds that make the most notable essential oil in aromatherapy today. There are roughly two thousand genera in the Rosa family, including hibiscus, roses, apricots, cherries, and plums.

The Persian scientist Avicenna was credited for discovering steam distillation in the 11th century, just to produce rosewater, a product he was so entranced with, and he wrote an entire book on it. His search for the perfect way to preserve roses and study their healing effects lay the groundwork for what would become aromatherapy.

The magic of rose is manifold. It has long been associated with love, but this is not the only power the rose holds. Rose has been associated with healing as long as it has with love and the romantic arts. A historic charm for treating victims of lightning strikes involved crushing roses and purslane together to make a poultice to treat the burns associated with lightning injuries. Since rose contains a large dose of vitamin C and can reduce redness, it stands to reason it would look quite magical to the healers of the time. Other sources conflate the rose with the magic of secrets.

Uses

Snip a healthy and firm rosebud an inch below the bulb of the stem. Thread a needle and pierce the stem of the rose halfway between its new end and the bud and hang to dry in a well-ventilated area (a moldy rose will not do). Once fully dry, bless in a manner appropriate to the traditions of the household. Use as a pendulum to divine secrets, love relationships, and issues of forgiveness, fidelity, and friendship.

The divinatory power of rose can be used for divination of all kinds. Scrying with rose is done a few ways:

- Place a drop of rose absolute in a dark-colored bowl of water and wait for images to appear.

- For an earthier form of scrying, fill a wooden bowl with rose petals, fresh or dried, and start tossing them to mix. This is a moving meditation, and moving for journeys, meditation, and scrying can put someone into a trance more rapidly than telling someone to sit still and wait for pictures to appear in their heads.

- For fire scrying, burn dried rose petals over incense charcoal to induce visions in the curls of smoke.

- For air scrying, place a drop of rose absolute in a water diffuser and watch the patterns created by the vapor.

Roses are bringers of good fortune, because roses were costly and could fetch a good price at a market for the wealthier set. Add a dried rose petal to your wallet to ensure the luck finds its way into the real world.

Roses have long been associated with love, lust, fertility, and fidelity. Wear a drop of diluted rose oil behind each ear to attract love and committed relationships. (With rose being largely diluted already, three drops of rose oil in a 1-ounce bottle of carrier is plenty.)

Historical references to roses and secrets abound. Several secret societies were said to have left roses on doorsteps to remind inhabitants of oaths they had made. Tell your secrets to a fresh rosebud and care for it until it starts to fade. Hang upside down to dry. Once completely dry, burn it in a fireplace or firesafe container. Sprinkle the ashes into a swiftly moving body of water to carry these cares far from you. Keep in mind, a burden shared is a burden halved. Tell someone you trust. It helps.

Because roses are a small, quiet bud that erupts into a riot of color and scent, they are associated with transformation. When the time comes that change is needed, anoint a white candle with diluted rose oil and burn on a Monday for an emotionally smooth transition. Rose also carries the magic of calm, harmony, and balance; it will help there as well.

Rose absolute is banishing for anxiety. Growing roses is therapeutic for some, but if plants only come to your home for end-of-life services, rose oil will do the trick beautifully. Add a drop of rose absolute to a water diffuser while slowly breathing in through the nose and out through the mouth. Repeat until peace is achieved and anxiety is banished for another day. Rose is also beneficial for removing the stress of family clashes.

To expand awareness outside oneself, meditate with rose. Turn off outside distractions, phones, television, etc. (Soothing music or drums are helpful for some, and not helpful for others. New age music works for some; classic rock works for me. Try out a few types of music and silence alternately to see what works. Noise-canceling headphones are also an option.) Place a drop of rose absolute in a water diffuser and close your eyes. While breathing slowly and evenly, in through the nose and out through the mouth, visualize your body. Find the limits of your physical form, where your skin ends and your aura begins. Now fill your aura with awareness from within. With each breath feel this bubble of awareness stretch and grow. This is a genuine sense, just as real as sight, sound, and smell, called proprioception. It is the link between awareness inside the body and the outside world. Developing this sense is beneficial not just to the well-being of the body (and shins, because furniture seems to have a mind of its own) but also of the world of magic around us. Proprioception is what allows us to feel the boundaries of the circles witches cast and the energies raised therein. By learning to stretch this mental ability, we can learn more about the world around us than we ever thought possible.

Rose is responsible not merely for banishing anxiety, but for the magic of hex breaking and banishing as a whole. To remove unwanted influences on self, home, family, or work, inscribe the influence on a black candle anointed with diluted rose oil and burn it on a Saturday.

Communication of a loving and whole variety is the hallmark of rose. In order to calm household tensions and allow for open, honest, and loving communication, diffuse rose oil or rosewater in the space where the discussion is to take place, up to thirty minutes beforehand. Rose also helps to calm and center emotional responses.

Producing Oils for Public Consumption

Always alert people to the contents of anointing oils, as even the gentlest essential oils can have people who are allergic. Do not take it personally; these are things we are born with, and allergies can come on at any point in life. If someone is allergic to a particular oil, offer charged water as an alternative.

Courage and rose go hand in hand. With the added energy of love and friendship, diffuse rose to bolster nerves when looking to move from friendship to love interest, or when wanting to take romantic relationships to the next level. Rose reminds us that not only are we capable, but we deserve good and beautiful things in our lives. Rose also carries the energy of compassion, so even if the answer is no the relationship will survive. Rose also instills confidence, so give it a go.

Rose has been associated with goddesses for as long as they have had a name. Using rose absolute as a consecration oil is one of the oldest uses of this blessed flower. Place a drop of diluted rose oil on objects or people to consecrate them before ritual.

As anyone who has ever handled a rose can tell you, roses have thorns. This makes rose a befitting oil for protection work. It is grounded in love and friendship, so it is particularly well suited to protecting loved ones and friends. If a friend or loved one has asked for protection magic, write their name on a brown candle (to ground anything potentially nasty coming their way) and anoint with diluted rose oil. Burn the rose on a Sunday.

Stuck between two suitors? Have an argument with a friend that doesn't make sense? Rose helps to provide emotional clarity. Diffuse rose absolute while puzzling out issues (making a good list of pros and cons also never hurts).

Rose is the scent of spiritual awakening. Making a daily practice to anoint the third eye with diluted rose oil and concentrating on the breath for a few moments can make a considerable difference in the quality of spiritual connection. Colloquial wisdom states that it takes twenty-one days to form a new habit; try this practice for twenty-one days and record that journey. See if there are spiritual changes that benefit further practice.

Roses come in such a variety of colors, shapes, and scents that they have been associated with creativity, especially for artists. If you're daydreaming of your next big project, show, or concept, diffuse a drop of rose absolute to allow those creative juices to flow. Alternately, use diffusing salts or an aroma necklace if your space is not conducive to a water diffuser.

Those thorns that rose is rocking aren't just for pricking thumbs. They can also be used to unblock stuck energy. If a chakra feels blocked, anoint the spot with diluted rose oil. A roller bottle can be useful if you're drawing sigils, or symbols of power, on a blocked energy spot. If the energetic block is in another area of life outside the body, write it on a white candle (purity) and burn it on a Sunday (solar transformation, luck) to transmute that stuck energy into something useful.

Kid Gloves Spell

Rose is not some wilting hothouse flower; it is potent, powerful, and carries its own thorns capable of protecting it. Because rose comes armed, it must be handled with gentleness.

To encourage others to treat you with gentleness, take a piece of paper and draw a figure. It can be a self-portrait or a gingerbread man. Name it after yourself or the name of your child. Give it a deactivation date (a birthdate can be helpful).

Using rose anointing oil in a roller bottle, draw an outline around the figure, completely enclosing it. It can be close to the skin, like an aura, or a large personal space bubble—that's a personal choice. Then inscribe the poppet's name on a pink candle and anoint it with the same rose oil. Burn the candle on a Monday (emotional well-being).

Rosewater

Those who grew up with cartoon movies of princesses and faerie tales will remember the story of Briar Rose and her beauty. The beauty magic of rose can be found easily in drugstore and upscale beauty brands. Rose removes redness and imparts vitamin C to the skin, and gives it a dewy finish. Consider making your own rosewater for skincare from organic roses. Just add the fresh rosewater to a spray bottle, mist the face, and gently wipe with a cotton round to remove excess oil and dirt.

The uses for rosewater are endless: Mist pillow before bed for a cool oasis and sweet dreams. Remind loved ones to act with honor by diffusing rosewater in a space during negotiations. Avert misfortune by diffusing rosewater in the home for an energetic spritzing up.

You will need two dozen roses (or more!)

Two heat-resistant bowls of similar size

Stockpot with lid

Distilled water

Ice

This is an easy home demonstration of water distilling. Place the first bowl face down in the bottom of the stockpot. Start removing the rose petals from the stems. The perfect roses are heavily scented. It is more important that the roses smell beautiful than look beautiful. Discount bin roses after Valentine's Day are fine, as long as they are not moldy. If using commercial roses, do not use this rosewater internally; there is no way of knowing how recently the roses were exposed to chemical sprays. Source organic roses for cosmetic purposes. Placing the rose petals inside the stockpot, keep filling the pot with rose petals until they are the level of the initial bowl.

Place the second bowl upright on top of the base of the first bowl. There may be room for a few roses at this point; use your best judgment. Fill the stockpot with water until it touches the bottom of the topmost bowl. Make sure no water gets into the top bowl. Place the stockpot's lid upside down on the pot. This will make a bowl for the ice to sit on. Add enough ice to fill the lid and keep it cool. Turn the heat on medium and watch the magic.

What's happening? The water is heating up with the rose petals, getting them to release their volatile oils. They will be released in the steam. The steam will rise and encounter the lid, filled with ice. The iced lid is cooler than the hot steam inside the pot and it will condense on the lid and drip into the topmost bowl to collect. Try not to disturb the lid too often; it is letting out steam. Once the bowl is filled, turn the heat off and allow the rosewater in the bowl to cool. Dump the cooked rose petals in the compost after it has cooled.

Add 1 teaspoon of 100-proof vodka (or 1 teaspoon of witch hazel, which is perfectly lovely for the skin) as a preservative and bottle the rosewater in sterilized containers (boil them or use the heated wash-and-dry setting on the dishwasher). Stores in the refrigerator for two to three weeks.

Rose Prayer Beads

The word *rosary* derives from Middle English and means "rose garden." Monks used to make beads from the rose bushes kept in monastic gardens, and now you can too. These beads can become a beloved family heirloom.

Two dozen roses (minimum)

Water or rosewater

Rose absolute (*Rosa damascena*)

Straight pins

Foam board

Optional: rusty iron nails

Harvest petals daily during rose blooming season. Alternatively, use organically grown roses from a florist, starting with two dozen. Cut out the white of the petal, if it has some, where it attaches to the flower.

Place petals in a cast-iron skillet or nonreactive pan with just enough water/rosewater to cover the petals. If you're using iron nails, add them to the pan now. (The iron helps produce a dark color in the beads. Look for masonry nails in the hardware store or use old nails—the rustier, the better.)

Turn the stove on the lowest setting possible. Stir rose petals occasionally and go about your day. Leave the heat on for a few hours at a time to remove the moisture and break the cell wall in the rose petals. The longer the heat can be left on, the faster the process.

Pick more rose petals every day through the two-week bloom time. Add them to the pan and, if necessary, add more water to just barely cover the petals.

Once the mixture resembles a thick clay, add 8 to 10 drops rose absolute and stir thoroughly. Start rolling beads, keeping a uniform size. They should be larger than a pea, but smaller than a lima bean. Remember, they will shrink as they dry. Repeat until none of the rose petal clay remains.

Once you've rolled all of your beads, stick a pin through each one and stick the pin to the foam board. This will facilitate even drying. Turn each bead on its pin after 24 hours, repeating daily, to ensure beads don't stick to the pin. Wetting your fingers with diluted rose oil will keep beads from cracking or sticking to your fingers. Beads can take a few weeks to dry, depending on temperature and moving air. When they're finally dry and ready, string beads as desired, for prayer or meditation. Consider stringing together with myrrh (*Commiphora myrrha*) beads for fragrance and the Divine. Even after the beads are dry, they will retain the scent of rose for decades to come.

Rosemary

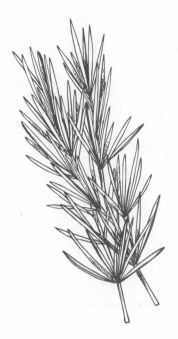

Scientific name: *Rosmarinus officinalis*

Botanical family: Lamiaceae

Origin: France, United States

Source of plant's oil: Leaves

Evaporation: Middle note

Scent description: Crisp, herbal, camphoraceous, medicinal, sweet

Scent impact: Improve clarity of thought

Magical Correspondences

Application: Diffuse, topical with dilution

Element: Fire

Day: Sunday

Magical uses: Purification, mental clarity, confidence, good luck

Planet: Sun

Astrological sign: Leo

Suggested crystal: Chrysocolla—ruled by Virgo: Encourages balanced, clear communication without being hindered by emotion

Deity/spirit: Athena, Greek goddess of wisdom, handicraft, and strategic war

Warnings

Herbs high in 1,8 cineole should not be used on or around children under five, as they can result in suffocation due to paralyzing of autonomic functions. Do not use if you have high blood pressure or epilepsy. Avoid during pregnancy. Possible skin irritant; use in low dilutions.

Herbal Lore

It is the herb Shakespeare called "the herb of remembrance." The Latin binomial tells one of the origin stories of this spicy member of the mint family: *Rosmarinus* means "dew of the sea," as one of this blue-flowered plant's origin stories involves the plant springing up where ocean water touched fertile soil.

Where rosemary flourishes, the woman rules.

—Traditional saying

Rosemary was often mixed with juniper and burned over charcoal to cleanse temple spaces of evil spirits throughout the Mediterranean.

Uses

Rosemary is a mark of character. If you are invoking the character of a person to make the correct choice, carve their name into a white candle and anoint it with diluted rosemary oil (1 drop rosemary essential oil in a 10 ml roller bottle filled with carrier oil). Burn the candle on a Sunday or at the full moon.

Confidence is sexy. To imbue yourself with winning confidence (not cockiness), wear a drop of rosemary essential oil in an aroma locket or place a dot of 1 percent diluted rosemary oil behind your ears. (Discontinue if irritation develops.) Bonus: rosemary also imparts courage.

Consecration has long been a duty of rosemary. Burning the dried leaves over charcoal for purification is one of the first recorded uses of this herb. Diffuse a drop or two of rosemary essential oil in a water diffuser to make a space sacred. Anoint ritual tools or sacred items with diluted rosemary oil (use with care on finished surfaces, as the oil can damage the finish).

Intellectual ability, quick thinking, and rational thought are determined uses of rosemary. Rosemary's reputation with thought and memory is so ingrained into societal memories that scientists have studied the folk properties of rosemary's memory boosting as a treatment for Alzheimer's. The current studies did not bear fruit, unfortunately. But diffusing rosemary during study periods and then carrying a tissue scented with a drop of rosemary essential oil during exams can help trigger sense memories associated with the study session.

Courage is a fiery side effect of working with this thought-boosting essential oil. When courage is needed, carry a sprig of rosemary in your pocket or a handkerchief with a drop of rosemary essential oil on it. A sprig of rosemary pinned to a suit lapel not only makes a dashing boutonnière but also benefits its wearer with courage, calm, and good luck.

The fire of rosemary is also adept at bringing things to an end, peacefully and at the correct time. Diffuse rosemary while writing out the ending desired (it can be in letter form or simply a single word). Physically writing it down will narrow the focus of the working. If it is safe to do so, place the paper beneath a black or white candle anointed with diluted rosemary oil and burn the candle on a Saturday. Added benefit: rosemary is the master at soothing a broken heart.

Good luck is on the horizon with any solar herb, but especially rosemary. The fire of this pine doppelgänger burns away negativity, leaving room for only good luck to pour in to fill the void. Inscribe a gold candle with "good luck" or other symbols and anoint it. Burn the candle on a Sunday.

Happiness is merely a drop away. Rosemary relieves anxiety, restores balance, and banishes fatigue to fight the feelings of sluggishness that a depressive state can bring. Diffuse a drop of rosemary in a 100 ml water diffuser while making a list, mental or physical, of all the things that bring joy. Keep this list handy for times when you are feeling down.

Samhain (pronounced SOW-en) is the festival remembering and honoring our beloved dead. It takes place starting at sunset on October 31, Halloween. If you desire a visit from a beloved family member who has gone across the veil, wear or carry a sprig of rosemary on Halloween day, and by the evening their spirit will be apparent.

Rosemary has a penchant for healing wild animals. Casting spells to help heal wild animals is noble; just do not harm yourself or the animal by trying to treat a wild animal without proper certifications and training. In many instances, it is also illegal. Call the local wildlife extension or wild animal rescue and follow their directions. A cornered wild animal is likely to strike out at perceived threats. Use caution.

Rosemary's use in purification and consecration rituals makes it a natural ally for banishing work of all kinds. Its history of increasing strength is also useful for banishing work. If someone or something needs to go, carve the person's name or the object to be banished into a black candle and anoint it with rosemary oil. Burn the candle on a Saturday.

The mind is too beautiful to waste. To stir thoughts, be uplifted, invoke happy memories, and release traumatic memories, diffuse rosemary essential oil while visualizing those traumatic memories on paper being torn to shreds and thrown into a volcano. Disempower the painful memories to be relieved of the weight of them and be transformed. Mental stability will follow like rain after clouds.

Rosemary is traditionally associated with happy marriages. Brides would weave wreaths and crowns to be worn during the wedding ceremony, and bundles of orange flowers and rosemary would be carried as bridal bouquets to bless the union. To invoke the magic of happy marriages, diffuse rosemary while engaging in a sweet night in, enjoying a dinner for two, or sharing a hobby with your partner.

Let go of nervousness, anxiety, restlessness, and nightmares with rosemary. Diffuse a drop or two of rosemary essential oil when it's time for a time out, up to thirty minutes before bed to banish nightmares, or to encourage rational thought. As an added benefit, rosemary can help you remember pleasant or prophetic dreams.

Meditation is facilitated by members of the mint family, and rosemary is no exception. Whether you're embarking on a guided journey of self-discovery or the centering of a blank slate, diffusing rosemary can benefit any meditative practice.

Hex-Breaking Spray

Busting hexes is easy with any member of the mint family. Let the strong medicinal scent of rosemary remind would-be hexes who is boss. Jinxes and curses do not stand a chance.

1 teaspoon witch hazel

3 drops rosemary essential oil (*Rosmarinus officinalis*) for hex breaking

Add witch hazel to a 2-ounce spray bottle of dark glass or number 1 plastic. Add rosemary essential oil to the witch hazel, cap, and shake. Unscrew the lid and fill the rest of the way with cool water. Cap and shake again.

Walk counterclockwise around the outside of the home, spraying the exterior so no hexes can cross the magical threshold created. If you live in an apartment, condo, or townhouse, spray the interior of your space. If family, roommates, or your spouse look concerned, this spray can also be used as a natural fabric refresher. (Just test a small portion of the fabric beforehand for colorfastness.) Use the remainder as a hand wash to keep nasty magic from following you home. (I highly recommend this practice to ghost hunters to ensure that nothing nasty comes home with them.)

Rosemary's Venusian associations were mentioned above, with wedding blessings, but that's not all. Rosemary is beneficial for work involving keeping a partner faithful, stirring passions that have waned, and blessing all those involved in the relationship. To remind a lover of promised fidelity, draw a heart on the bottom of their shoes (the ones worn the most) with diluted rosemary oil.

Protection is the flip side of the hex-breaking coin, and rosemary is a potent protection partner. Make protection sachets for loved ones to carry in their purse, book bag, briefcase, and more by filling muslin tea bags with dried rosemary. Anoint with a drop of rosemary essential oil and let the bags charge beneath the full moon. Distribute to loved ones for protection.

Along with the other mental powers purported by rosemary scholars, the power of wisdom is a key use. When difficult decisions are required, ask Athena for the wisdom to see the best course of action. Light a gray candle (said to be the color of Her eyes) and burn on a Monday. Rosemary is also associated with increase, so expand those thoughts and minds.

Comfort Bath

Take time to seek the comfort you need with this bath salt featuring rosemary.

Place 1 cup salt in a glass bowl and top with 3 drops rosemary essential oil. Combine by stirring well with a wooden spoon (only used for aromatherapy). Add desired amount of bath salts to a warm running bath. Allow the salt to purify the offending issue while deriving comfort from the rosemary's scent.

Effective communication is the foundation of any successful relationship, romantic or fraternal. If communication becomes muddy, diffuse rosemary for up to one half hour before the other party arrives to talk out the issue over tea or coffee. (See tea recipe below.)

Among the mental powers of rosemary, improved concentration and focus are at the top of the list. When focus is paramount, diffuse a drop of rosemary essential oil. If you are in an office environment that does not allow for diffusers, carry a tissue with a drop of rosemary essential oil on it, or (gently) inhale directly from the bottle once an hour. Do not use direct inhalation too frequently, though, as dizziness and nausea can occur.

Creativity is within reach. Rosemary will unlock any blocks to creativity that may exist and increase focus until the project is complete. Add a drop of rosemary oil to an aroma locket to power the creative juices. Rosemary also brings inspiration.

Not only is rosemary associated with bringing visions of the deceased, but burning dried rosemary or diffusing rosemary while talking to loved ones on the other side can help carry messages to them.

The courage and focus mentioned earlier that rosemary possesses can also encourage determination. When lines are drawn in the sand, rosemary is the one holding the line. When determination is called for, burn a yellow candle on a Tuesday to ensure wishes are heeded victoriously.

Friendship is a cherished gift. If new friendships are desired, burn dried rosemary leaves over incense charcoal while a wish for new beneficial friendships is made. The energy of honesty will help ensure that new friends are both truthful and of pure intention.

Hang rosemary over the threshold to prevent evil from entering the home.

Intuition is nurtured by rosemary. Attempt scrying with rosemary in three ways:

1. Place a drop of rosemary essential oil in a dark bowl of water for water scrying.

2. Burn dried rosemary leaves over incense charcoal for air scrying.

3. Combine water and air scrying: add a drop of rosemary essential oil to a water diffuser and allow the vapor to induce a trancelike state conducive to intuitive insight.

Rosemary Remembrance Tea

An herbal tea to drink and remember fondly.

2 teaspoons dried rosemary (*Rosmarinus officinalis*) for courage, release, strength, wisdom

1 teaspoon dried lemongrass (*Cymbopogon citratus*) for honesty, fidelity, calm

2 teaspoons dried peppermint (*Mentha piperita*) for clarity, healing, happiness

Blend the herbs and store in an airtight container away from sunlight until ready to use.

Boil water and place 1 to 2 teaspoons of tea in a reusable tea filter. Place the filter in a mug and pour boiled water over. Wait 5 minutes before removing herbs from tisane. (This beverage is not technically tea without *Camellia sinensis*.) Sweeten with sugar or honey, if desired, and enjoy slowly and quietly, remembering.

Samhain (Faux) Sourdough

Bake this for loved ones, bring it to a potluck, or leave it out for offerings. (Makes excellent pizza dough as well.)

2 to 3 sprigs rosemary (*Rosmarinus officinalis*) for clarity, transformation, honoring the dead, seeing ghosts, banishing sadness

1 cup self-rising flour

1 cup Greek yogurt

1 to 2 teaspoons olive oil

Optional: ½ teaspoon minced garlic for protection

Preheat oven to 350° Fahrenheit (177 degrees Celsius).

Pour olive oil into a custard cup and add garlic, if desired. Stir and set aside.

Add Greek yogurt to a mixing bowl and slowly incorporate self-rising flour until mixed. Knead another minute until well incorporated.

Roll out dough on a floured working space into a flatbread. Transfer to a baking sheet or stone.

Brush top of the dough with the olive oil. Strip the rosemary leaves from the stem and sprinkle on top of the dough. Bake 18 to 20 minutes or until golden brown.

Mabon Memories

Use this blend during harvest celebrations.

4 drops rosemary essential oil (*Rosmarinus officinalis*) for consecration, confidence, balance, blessings

11 drops benzoin essential oil (*Styrax tonkinensis*) for calming, harmony, inspiration, peace, wisdom

3 drops May Chang essential oil (*Litsea cubeba*) for meditation, prayer, strength, renewal, calm

25 drops neroli essential oil (*Citrus aurantium*) for protection, releasing negative emotions, defense against psychic attack, sleep, shielding

Blend all oils in a 2 ml bottle and diffuse synergy before harvest festivals, rituals, and parties. Can be used at Mabon, Thanksgiving, and gatherings of extended family to keep the peace and renew connections among family and friends. Add 2 drops of synergy to a 10 ml roller bottle and fill with carrier oil for anointing candles for magic involving family harmony, religious renewal, and worship.

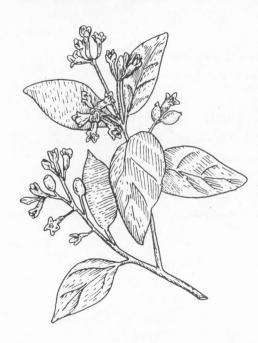

Sandalwood

Scientific name: *Santalum album* (white sandalwood); *Pterocarpus santalinus* (red sandalwood)

Botanical family: Santalaceae

Origin: India

Source of plant's oil: Bark

Evaporation: Base note

Scent description: Sweet, dark, woody

Scent impact: Ground emotional disturbances

Magical Correspondences

Application: Diffuse, dilute, topical application

WHITE SANDALWOOD

Element: Water

Day: Monday

Magical uses: Healing, nurturing, spirituality

Planet: Moon

Astrological sign: Cancer

Suggested crystal: Lapis lazuli—ruled by Sagittarius: ushers seekers into the mystical realms

Deity/spirit: Li Shizhen, Chinese God of Herbal Medicine

RED SANDALWOOD

Element: Fire

Day: Sunday

Magical uses: Love, protection, sensuality, sexuality

Planet: Sun

Astrological sign: Leo

Suggested crystal: Snakeskin agate—ruled by Scorpio: reminds us of the joy of living

Deity/spirit: Eir, who appears in the Poetic Eddas—provides women's medicine and mercy

HERBAL LORE

Sandalwood has a medicinal use history as long as its magical one. Ayurvedic medicine uses it to treat fevers, melancholy, peptic discomfort, and septic skin conditions. As many countries are cracking down on the export of this precious oil, it is getting more common to find adulterated, traded, and false oils. Sandalwood already diluted for use will be more readily available than the essential oil. When selecting a sandalwood to work with, buy the smallest amount allowed from a few companies and quality test them using the methods discussed in Appendix C: Testing Your Essential Oils for Quality and Purity. Work with them. See which oils produce results.

White sandalwood and red sandalwood are both used magically. White sandalwood is less fragrant than its red counterpart but has the same magical uses. While some magical texts assign different properties to the white versus the red sandalwood being offered, for this book it is okay to use them interchangeably. Keep in mind that sandalwood is a precious tree. As the tree grows, the red of the wood is bleached by the sun, leaving only the heartwood a ruddy red-brown. The heartwood of the sandalwood is used for distilling and will yield a high-quality oil with a yellowish tinge that will be expensive.

USES

Due to the increase in poaching sandalwood trees and strict export laws, ethical growing practices have flourished in countries like Australia where Australian sandalwood (*Santalum spicatum*) has started making up the lion's share of the market. For ethically sourced sandalwood, consider Australian sandalwood an aromatic replacement. As it is a very closely related species, it will carry the same correspondences, without the moral and ethical dilemmas of sourcing materials legally. The largest sustainable sandalwood farm in Australia is roughly three times the size of France and is heavily regulated by the Australian government to ensure standards of practice.

Sandalwood is an antianxiety essential oil. Diffuse a drop in a 100 ml water diffuser while taking slow, deep breaths to help overcome momentary struggles with anxiety.

Expand awareness outside the body and reach with those psychic senses. Sandalwood excels at helping to expand awareness beyond our day-to-day world. Astral travel is aided by sandalwood's properties of psychic development. It increases focus, benefits meditation practices, and clears the mind of the excess debris that accumulates during the day. Diffuse the mind while visualizing a blank slate. Breathe slowly and deeply for several minutes before attempting astral travel or divination.

Perform banishing magic at the drop of a hat. Sandalwood not only banishes negativity and unwanted feelings of loneliness, fear, and depression, it brings clarity to otherwise murky situations. Place 1 drop sandalwood essential oil in a 2 ml bottle and fill with carrier oil of choice. Cap and shake. This anointing oil can be used for banishing magic with ease. Select a colored candle for the banishing magic at hand. (See chapter 2 for suggestions on color magic.) Anoint the candle with the diluted sandalwood oil, tell it what needs to go, and light it, preferably during a waning moon or on a Saturday.

All of the base oils, especially the dark and woody ones, are beneficial for grounding, centering, and calming work. Sandalwood is especially beneficial to this work because of its associations of spirituality and consecration. It helps remind us that we are all spiritual beings who deserve love and respect. For grounding, centering, or consecration work, anoint ritual tools with diluted sandalwood oil (beware, as oils can damage wooden finishes). Anoint yourself as well, if desired; diluted sandalwood is skin safe. (Patch test to check for allergies first, and discontinue use if irritation occurs.) Sandalwood also encourages harmony within the self and with others.

Help a loved one recover after surgery. Charge a 2 ml bottle filled with 1 drop of sandalwood essential oil and carrier oil. Present this healing potion to the person recovering. They can place a drop behind each ear and on pulse points to remind them of the healing energy of sandalwood. The emollient effects of the oil can be used to minimize scar tissue after any surgical wounds have healed completely. Note: Never apply an essential oil to an open wound. And do not apply undiluted essential oils to the skin. Chemical burns can result.

Nurture the spark of creative madness that lives within everyone. If a particular project is desired, anoint a yellow (thought) candle with diluted sandalwood oil and burn on a Wednesday (communication) or Friday (beauty and the arts).

Sandalwood is an antidepressant and can work in concert with professional interventions such as talk therapy and medication if needed. For a mood booster, diffuse a drop of sandalwood essential oil during meditation or while taking care of daily tasks.

To settle chaotic or disturbing dreams, diffuse sandalwood oil up to a half hour before bedtime for gentle dreams of comfort and safety. Sandalwood also brings balance and calm.

To gain freedom from an untenable situation, anoint a candle with the name of the person or situation from which freedom is needed. Burn on a Saturday (endings) to cut those ties. If the situation merits, consider involving law enforcement, as situations can be unpredictable. If the offender is a stalker, ring the property on which your home resides in dried mugwort to keep them from discovering the location of your residence.

Emotional growth is not easy, but it's a worthwhile goal. Emotional growth is more than learning when to face our inner demons. It can positively impact every interaction with friends, family, coworkers, and acquaintances. It results in a lower stress response and lowers blood pressure. Diffuse sandalwood essential oil while engaging in positive mantras such as "others' reactions and opinions are their own." Sandalwood also encourages emotional stability.

Desiring some spiritual guidance? Hoping a teacher will come along and explain the things that are happening? Grab a purple candle (the divine) and anoint it with diluted sandalwood oil. If a teacher is hoped for, snag a blue candle for trust, intuition, and guidance and anoint it with diluted sandalwood oil. Say a few words describing the wish or need before lighting. Sandalwood also carries the magic of manifestation.

Focus and concentration running thin? Diffuse sandalwood to calm and center long enough to focus on the task at hand.

Legal battles are nerve wracking, unsettling, and costly. Fortunately, justice is a delightful perk of working with sandalwood. To gain a fair judge and ask for blessings on the court case, write "bless me" on a white candle (purity of thought) and anoint it with sandalwood oil. Traditional Just Judge oils also contain bergamot, so add a drop of bergamot essential oil too, if desired.

All kinds of professionals need inspiration in their fields—not just painters, sculptors, and authors. Diffuse sandalwood while clearing the mind of excess chatter. By clearing out the voices of grocery lists, personal and professional duties, and deadlines, we make room for inspiration to flourish. If diffusion is not possible in the current environment, place a drop of the essential oil on a tissue and breathe deeply and slowly while smelling the oil. Aroma lockets are also handy in these situations. Sandalwood is an excellent choice anytime clearing the mind is needed—especially of negativity or nervousness.

Interested in discovering the parts left behind in a past life? Reach for sandalwood. Not only can sandalwood aid when journeying to past lives, but it also encourages psychic development and relaxation, and imbues sacred protection from the Divine.

Seeking the truth on an important matter? Burn red sandalwood chips over incense charcoal while meditating and watching the smoke. Allow the mind to drift and await messages from the Divine, or spirit guides.

Sandalwood is a potent hex breaker and uncrossing oil, and as it carries the energies of success not much can stand up to it. Anoint a black candle with diluted sandalwood oil and burn it on a Saturday during the waning moon.

Do you have a desire to explore a new spiritual path, or develop a deeper relationship with your current one? Visualizations with sandalwood can help uncover the innermost parts of the psyche. Carve your desire into a white or purple candle and anoint it with sandalwood oil. Burn the candle on a Monday.

To encourage new business opportunities, anoint a green (money) or gold (luck, prosperity) candle with diluted sandalwood oil and burn the candle on a Thursday (protected growth).

Protection, both spiritual and physical, is the trademark of sandalwood. For physical threats, sandalwood negates their influence and brings the law to aid. In the case of spiritual protection, sandalwood is said to cast out demons, bring the blessings of the universe, and release fears, sorrows, and obstacles.

Sandalwood carries the energies of success, luck, and wishes. When things seem out of reach, turn to sandalwood. Anoint a yellow or gold candle with diluted sandalwood oil and burn it on a Sunday.

Big, Bad Be Gone Oil

This powerful blend is well suited for exorcism and protection magic.

4 drops Australian sandalwood essential oil (*Santalum spicatum*) for protection, exorcism

3 drops sweet basil essential oil (*Ocimum basilicum*) for protection, exorcism

4 drops lavender essential oil (*Lavandula angustifolia*) for longevity, purification, protection

4 teaspoons carrier oil

Blend oils in a small glass or number 1 plastic bottle and roll it between your hands, or shake gently. Add carrier oil and shake or roll again to blend. Apply this oil to your pulse points for protection.

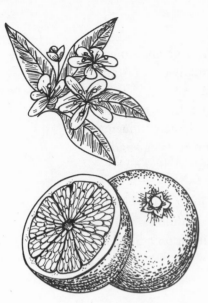

Tangerine (aka Mandarin)

Scientific name: *Citrus reticulata*

Botanical family: Rutaceae

Origin: China, United States, South America

Source of plant's oil: Peels

Evaporation: Top note

Scent description: Sweet, citrus, light, tangy, fruity

Scent impact: Attain joy

Magical Correspondences

Application: Diffuse, direct inhalation, topical with care

Element: Fire

Day: Sunday

Magical uses: Purification, protection, clarity, lifting mood

Planet: Sun

Astrological sign: Leo

Suggested crystal: Larimar—ruled by Leo: removes self-limiting behavioral patterns

Deity/spirit: Sekhmet, ancient Egyptian goddess of the sun, war, and healing

Warnings

Patch test diluted oil, and take care given citrus's acidic nature. Do not use with dilutions greater than 2.5 percent without supervision.

Uses

Place a drop of tangerine essential oil in an aroma locket to bring a joyful spring to each step.

Tangerine governs the magic of calm, cool, and collected. To restore calm to a chaotic home, anoint a candle (orange is an uplifting and thoughtful color) with 1 drop tangerine essential oil in a 2 ml bottle filled with carrier oil. Burn on a Sunday or Friday.

Whether you're looking to clear away mental fog or bring clarity to a situation, tangerine is ideal. Diffuse a drop of tangerine essential oil while mulling over an issue, thinking on paper (pro and con lists are well suited to this), or meditating for an emotional boost, calm thinking, and clarity on the subject.

To create beneficial dreams, banish nightmares and night terrors, and settle sleep patterns, diffuse tangerine essential oil up to thirty minutes before retiring for the evening.

Hospitality is religion in many cultures. To boost your energy before an event, as well as relieve the associated stress and increase the bonds of friendship among those attending, diffuse tangerine essential oil throughout preparations on the day of and throughout the event. It will be a subtle fragrance note, and future encounters with the fragrance will remind partygoers of the enjoyment they shared.

Inspiration is the bread and butter for creative people of many jobs, cultures, and aspirations. Creative pursuits do not fall only under the auspices of artists. To increase the inspiration and creative flow, diffuse tangerine essential oil in studios, offices, and workspaces.

You've probably heard the saying, "Make hay while the sun shines." With the sun to bless endeavors, little can stand against it. When hex breaking and uncrossing, working in the light of the full sun can boost those energies. Solar herbs like tangerine are the perfect addition to any uncrossing work, even on a cloudy day. To cut ties that bind, uncross a threshold, or break a hex, anoint a black candle (for uncrossing, hex breaking) with diluted tangerine oil and burn on a Saturday (endings).

Tangerine is not only banishing toward hexes or curses, it has a beneficial use for banishing negativity as well. It does not just center the self; it uplifts and supports emotional well-being, calmness, and a positive outlook. Diffuse tangerine essential oil when a mood boost is needed to get through the day.

Having established that tangerine is capable of instilling calm, it should be noted that the reverse is also true. Because it instills calm, tangerine is appropriately suited to banishing nervousness, anxiety, and fear. Wear a drop of tangerine essential oil in an aroma locket to keep negative feelings at bay all day long. If an aroma locket is not in the cards, carry a tissue with a drop of tangerine essential oil on it. (Handkerchiefs are not recommended, as the dark orange oil will stain fabric.)

If a spell, charm, or talisman is in need of a little extra oomph, tangerine essential oil can provide extra power. Add dried tangerine peel with a drop of tangerine essential oil on it to mojo bags for a citrus boost. Anoint talismans regularly with diluted tangerine oil to keep the intention going.

Along with the light that burns in protection, those same solar associations are purifying. Allow the energy of the sun to purify the self, home, or work of anything that either no longer serves or never did serve you. Diffuse tangerine while planning lists of items to purge from a home. Calming and purifying traits make tangerine the perfect essential oil to diffuse while talking out an argument and making up.

Tangerine not only aids uncrossing or hex breaking, it is excellent as a defensive oil as well. Armor your home, car, self, and office with tangerine essential oil in diffusers to create a wall against any outside threats.

Practicing trance skills for journeying, divination, or other magic? Tangerine can help. An easy-to-use trance tool is the diffuser. Place 100 ml water in the well per drop of tangerine oil. Once it has been turned on, watch the water vapor. Unfocus your eyes, and allow your mind to drift and images to appear and pass by.

Quick and Dirty Prosperity Spell

As with other solar herbs, prosperity is a drop away. For a quick and dirty prosperity spell, grab a piece of flash paper, a birthday candle, and diluted tangerine oil. Write the prosperous need on the flash paper. 1" x 2" booklets can be had in local magic supply shops. (Stage magicians use it for a flash of fire in the palm of the hand without heat, smoke, or ash.) Anoint the birthday candle with diluted tangerine oil. Light the birthday candle, and feel free to say a few words. As the candle burns, think of the need burning in the back of your mind. As the candle nears the end of its wick, touch the flame to the paper and let go. (Feel free to do a trial run with the flash paper first if you're nervous about the idea of fire in your hand.) The flash of fire releases the energy of the burning candle quickly and easily and allows you to soon go on about the day.

Citrus Room Spray for Protection

Protection magic is the herald for many solar deities. While uncrossing and hex breaking, it is also important to understand that the protective aspects of tangerine can make sure none of those issues can reattach. Whether or not tangerine is the oil used in hex breaking, or uncrossing, it is a strong protection herb. Place a teaspoon of the salt of choice in a glass bowl. Mix 3 drops of tangerine into the salt with a nonreactive implement, such as a wooden spoon. (Do not use aluminum, as it will react.) Add to a 2-ounce spray bottle and fill with warm water. Spray the outside of the home, or the interior walls if walls are shared with neighbors. Try to stick to the edges of the floors inside, as the spray could stain painted surfaces or carpet. Test carefully to avoid damage. See the entirety of the home enclosed in a bright orange ring that burns anything nasty directed toward the home.

Lovely Hostess

Diffuse this blend while preparing for a party or other social event.

6 drops tangerine essential oil (*Citrus reticulate*) for
hospitality, calm, clarity

1 drop ginger essential oil (*Zingiber officinale*) for energy,
beauty, power

5 drops petitgrain essential oil (*Citrus aurantium*) for self-
purification and energy

The energy of a host(ess) can make or break a gathering. Whether
you're hosting a coven gathering, a cocktail party, or an open circle
with close friends, the preparation can take a toll. Diffuse this energizing blend while tending the pre-gathering to-do list. Feel free to
keep it going once the guests arrive; they will be energized and happy
as well. And the next time they smell the delicate tangerine, they will
remember fondly the great time they had. Just don't be surprised
when you're asked to host again soon.

Getting to Know You

Diffuse this blend during the getting-to-know-you phase of new
romances and friendships.

5 drops tangerine essential oil (*Citrus reticulate*) for honesty,
calm, joy, protection

5 drops lavender essential oil (*Lavandula angustifolia*) for
secrets, centering, peace

10 drops sandalwood essential oil (*Santalum album*) for
wishes and honesty

Diffuse this to encourage honesty, banish nervousness, and create a
safe place for sharing secrets and bonding. Place 1 drop of the synergy in a 100 ml diffuser.

Vetiver or Vetivert

Scientific name: *Vetiveria zizanioides*

Botanical family: Poaceae

Origin: India, Haiti

Source of plant's oil: Roots

Evaporation: Base note

Scent description: Dark, resinous, grassy, earthy, sweet

Scent impact: Find grounding and beneficial coping mechanisms

Magical Correspondences

Application: Direct inhalation, diffuse, topical application with proper dilution

Element: Earth

Day: Friday

Magical uses: Grounding, aphrodisiac, commanding, hex breaking

Planet: Venus

Astrological sign: Taurus

Suggested crystal: Garnet—ruled by Virgo: a pledge to oneself, grounded self-love

Deity/spirit: Gaea, primordial goddess of the Earth

Warnings

Possible skin sensitizer. Use in dilutions below 2.5 percent.

Herbal Lore

Though vetiver essential oil is made from the roots of a member of the grass family, in ancient times the blades of grass were dried and burned to purify spaces and break curses laid on home, family, and self.

Due to vetiver's earthy smell, it has associations with money and prosperity, and has been sprinkled in cash drawers and coin purses to increase business in stores and markets for hundreds of years.

The Venusian connotations also make it popular in spells of sex, romance, love, and lust for all genders and orientations. In hoodoo, it is used not only for matters of love but also fidelity and faithfulness.

Because vetiver is a root, it has an abundance of the volatile oils that make this earthy, warm, and sensual smell. That makes it a marvelous addition to spells, charms, and mojo bags to increase the power, stability, and long-term effect of workings. Feed a charm bag monthly with a drop of vetiver essential oil to keep the working going.

Uses

Vetiver is an herb of passion, attraction, and sexuality. Unlike some of the floral essential oils that are associated with love, lust, and sex, vetiver is not dependent on the sex of the person using it, or the sex of the person desired. Vetiver is used in Venusian workings for all sexes, genders, and orientations.

Vetiver is a grounding herb that is attributed with the ability to strengthen, fill, and patch the aura. Think of it as a magical wall Spackle that can repair holes in the aura while strengthening existing structures. Holes in the aura can be caused by illness, trauma, soul loss, psychic vampirism, and magical sabotage. Problems in the auric field can be diagnosed by aura cameras, shamans, magical practitioners, and intuitives, and by sight or feel with practice. As with any kind of intuitive work, there are honest practitioners and there are charlatans; look for a practitioner with a good reputation, with clients you know. Rates are usually on par with bodywork such as massage and reiki.

Life making "hectic" seem like a leisurely stroll through the park? Vetiver can be utilized to restore balance. Diffuse vetiver while making a list of actionable items to reduce stress and increase calm. This grounding oil can bring peace and ground excess energy and chaotic vibrations. To slow the number of things the universe is throwing your way, anoint a brown candle (stability) with diluted vetiver oil (1 drop of vetiver essential oil in a 10 ml roller bottle filled with carrier oil) and burn during the dark moon or on a Monday.

The grounding aspects of vetiver make it an incredible ally for banishing work. Whereas a solar herb like orange can banish because it burns out the connections, vetiver grounds energies that need banishing to be transmuted by the earth. This makes vetiver befitting to work banishing grief, jealousy, and negativity. Diffusing vetiver is the fastest method toward any of these goals. If it is impractical to utilize a water diffuser, add a drop of vetiver essential oil to an aroma locket.

There comes a time when every business needs a boost, and the earthly connections of vetiver make it ideal for work in finance, success, money, and all matters of business. Working with vetiver essential oil, derived from roots, for business and financial matters leads to long-term and steady growth (vetiver's oil comes from its roots, rooting that success in the long term). Vetiver has been noted in magic for manifestation; therefore, if customers are needed, manifest them with vetiver. Anoint an orange (success) candle with diluted vetiver oil and burn it on a Sunday.

Vetiver also brings luck and is connected to the idea of wealth, rather than fast cash, due to its long-acting nature. It benefits finance not only in the immediate future but also in the long-term.

Court cases are stressful times. Allow magic to be the instrument for clarity, success, and fairness with vetiver. Wear an aroma locket with a drop of vetiver when seeing (and seeking) a lawyer, and during any hearings for the court case. It will provide strength and calm while reinforcing the fairness of the judge and the system.

The banishing aspects of vetiver as well as its ability to instill calm make it a strong choice for managing depression magically. Try diffusing a drop of vetiver essential oil in water to center, calm, and instill peace. Take care, though. Magic may bring agency and control, but it is no replacement for talk therapy, medications, or other professional interventions.

Because of its tendency to empower by banishing depression, and fortify emotions and the aura, vetiver is ideal for magic involving happiness. Vetiver blends well with grapefruit, so use these oils together to find happiness when days are dark and filled with doubt. Grapefruit is a solar herb and beneficial for magic involving lifting emotional burdens. Diffuse a drop of each in a water diffuser to be reminded of happy times and increase harmony and joy.

Vetiver's grounding aspects lead to cultivating discipline and focus. When on a deadline and pressure is mounting, diffuse vetiver to encourage focus and drive.

Vetiver is commanding and settling, and as such will remove obstacles to goals. If something is standing in the way of your goals, anoint a black candle with diluted vetiver oil and burn it on a Saturday during the waning moon for best effect.

Increase the security of your home by practicing banishing and protection magic that features vetiver. Not only is vetiver helpful with banishing, but in all of those tendencies to rid of the unwanted, vetiver is also an herb of protection. It forms a barrier between harmful energies and persons, and grounds energies that are not in our highest good. To protect from negative energies and people, wear a drop of vetiver essential oil in an aroma locket for portable protections. Use diluted vetiver oil to anoint doors, windows, and electrical and water inlets into the home, and the backs of mirrors. Feel free to inscribe the protective symbol of choice with the oil, or a simple circle for wholeness or a square for stability.

The calm that follows vetiver makes it an ideal companion for relaxation. Leave the stresses of the outside world behind. Diffuse vetiver during relaxing baths or meditation. Vetiver is not recommended for bath salts, however, as it has a potentially sensitizing effect on the skin.

Vetiver's ability to strengthen the aura is not its only outlet. It's also legendary for its physical strength. If you are dealing with a physical aliment, reach for vetiver. Those undergoing serious physical recovery, multiple broken bones, rehabilitation, or reconstruction will benefit from a strengthening oil. When physical therapy seems endless, the list of doctors daunting, or the pain never ending, diffuse vetiver to remember where the center lies and tap into the endless strength of the gods and the earth. Vetiver will also ground the emotional stresses that a long-term illness or recovery can heap upon an already stressed situation.

Protect homes, cars, and offices from thieves with vetiver oil. Instead of the protection of other herbs that could shield personal belongings but subject another to the fate averted, the magic of vetiver will ground the impulses that lead to the offensive behavior. Thieves prey on people for a variety of reasons. Contact with the magic of vetiver will dull the would-be thief's impulses long enough for him or her to consider the motivations for their actions and the potential implications.

The grounding intentions of vetiver also make it worthy for hex-breaking work. Threads of curses, hexes, and jinxes are transmuted by the earth, where they are grounded. The planet can handle those energies in a way that is harmless to it, whereas a person could be negatively affected.

Among the protective aspects of vetiver, it is important to note its use in magic for psychic protection. We all know someone who makes a five-minute conversation feel like two hours. Maybe we find ourselves avoiding their phone calls, and even turning around in the hallway when we see them coming, rather than engaging. Those are the symptoms of psychic vampirism, whether they understand what is happening or not. Many energy leeches have no understanding that this is the effect they have on others, and it is doubtful they would be able to correct the issue without work, dedication, and possibly therapy. In order to protect your psyche and your physical energy, wear a drop of vetiver essential oil in an aroma locket or carry a tissue that has a drop of the essential oil on it. (Handkerchiefs are not recommended due to the dark color of the oil staining the fabric.) If this person is a coworker, keep this tissue on hand for daily surprise encounters. If they are a frequent visitor to your space (home or office), diffuse vetiver oil if possible.

Regeneration is an indication of vetiver oil as well. If energetic stores are depleted, rely on vetiver to help restore and maintain both psychic and physical energetic levels. Vetiver is not a quick fix (for that, reach for a citrus oil, like grapefruit), but it will last longer. Create a blend of fast-acting and long-acting oils so relief starts working quickly, but has a sustained effect. Diffuse a drop of each oil when feeling emotionally and physically depleted.

Make the First Move Oil

Use this blend to show interest in a potential partner.

- 1 drop vetiver essential oil (*Vetiveria zizanioides*) for aphrodisiac and grounding
- 3 drops black pepper essential oil (*Piper nigrum*) for physical energy, courage
- 4 drops sweet orange essential oil (*Citrus sinensis*) for attraction, beauty, luck

This is designed as the oil equivalent of a "Do you like me? Check YES or NO" note. It will not interfere with anyone's free will; it is simply a flare signaling interest in situations where walking up to the intended and stating interest could be met with awkwardness, fear, or violence. If the person is also interested, they are free to make the first move.

Diffuse this oil as a signal to the universe that you are ready for love.

Anoint a red or pink candle with 1 drop of synergy in a 2 ml bottle filled with the carrier oil of your choice. Burn the candle on a Friday (love, beauty) during the waxing moon for best effect. This oil will not interfere with the free will of any persons. This is a flare, signaling interest. If the person is also interested, they are free to make the first move.

Lift Spirits, Gain Focus Oil

Use this blend to regain energy, focus, and insight.

- 5 drops vetiver essential oil (*Vetiveria zizanioides*) for increased focus, success

- 8 drops clary sage essential oil (*Salvia sclarea*) to combat depression and improve balance, wisdom

- 10 drops ylang-ylang essential oil (*Cananga odorata*) to raise vibrations and relax

Blend essential oils in a 2 ml bottle. Dilute 1 drop of synergy in a 2 ml bottle of carrier oil to anoint candles, charms, and talismans for emotional support and wisdom, and to raise the vibrations of the subject.

Botanical Divination   7

Divination is the means of attempting to discern information through an indirect, nontraditional method such as tarot, oracle cards, runes, scrying, tea leaf reading, pendulums, bibliomancy, palmistry, stone oracles, or other means. The oracle that you design can be a permanent one, such as a homemade deck of cards or stones, or single use, as with freshly carved rune staves.

DIVINATION METHODS OVERVIEW

There are many types of divination tools in the world, and you can create or use any of them to fit your needs.

Tarot

The earliest documented tarot cards date back to 1440 CE and have since spawned thousands of designs. In our digital age, you can even find tarot deck apps that bring the power of divination to your smartphone. The Fool's Dog is one such company that creates apps for witches and other divination enthusiasts. If you want to learn, there are decks for all, featuring classic artwork from masters like da Vinci, Klimt, and even Bosch, manga, playing card/tarot crossover decks, and more. Because the bulk of tarot decks keep within the same symbolism and closely mirror the artwork once the cards are understood, that language translates to most other decks. They're a permanent system, barring a tragic accident with your morning coffee or an open car window.

Tarot is an immensely popular and personal tool. Once someone has bonded with a particular deck they may forsake all others, and procure special storage solutions and the like. My dear friend Michael was once hit by a car while carrying his favorite deck and actually asked the first responders to pick up his scattered tarot cards before loading him into the ambulance to take him to the hospital.

Oracle Cards

Oracle cards have a similar personal touch, and you can learn a lot about someone if given the chance to peek into their cartomancy collection. Are they all nature-themed oracle decks? Are there only animal oracles? Perhaps their entire collection features the fae. The oracle systems are vastly different and deeply personal. While the tarot has a rich history and widespread symbolism to draw from, oracle systems are as different as night and day. One of my decks is simply detailed photographs of tumbled and raw gemstones. It speaks very deeply to me, but it might not make any sense to someone else. An oracle based on gorgeous cemetery headstones also exists. The point is that each person can find his or her own personality within an oracle. Conversely, you might use several oracles for the different types of personalities encountered while reading. For example, my dearest Peep, the matriarch of our clan, used to see a woman in her small, Italian, Baltimore neighborhood who read greeting cards instead of tarot cards. "Tarot cards are of the Devil," she'd say, "but greeting cards are of Hallmark." All of the older ladies in the neighborhood would save their couponing money to pay for their readings, and, word had it, she was never wrong.

Runes

Runes are, in my experience, a much more generalized tool. The fewer cards, stones, or other tools used in a divination method, the more general the messages are. Themes of wealth, strength, protection, cleansing, and the chaos of nature are all themes we can relate to. They're perfect for my one-a-day rune pull that helps me figure out a theme for the day, or tips me off to something to be aware of. Runes are now commonly made from stones of all types, but I prefer my wooden friends.

Scrying

Scrying is a type of divination involving gazing deeply into a surface in order to turn off the waking mind and tap into the subconscious mind. It is one of the easiest methods to set up, yet the hardest to employ for many folks. All you need is one of the elements—water, air, fire, or earth—and you've got your medium. The hard part is letting go of the conscious mind and allowing the images to appear to you. This may not happen right away; it depends on how much time and energy you've devoted in your life and practice to meditation. Some folks think simply willing images to appear will cause it to happen. This is simply not true.

GETTING INTO THE RIGHT FRAME OF MIND

Autostereograms, or "Magic Eye" images, are a series of books and artwork that allow the viewer to experience a three-dimensional picture in a two-dimensional space. The trick is that you cannot actually look for the 3-D image you hope to see; you have to look *through* the picture. In order to see, you have to un-focus your eyes.

This forced perspective relaxation has frustrated a lot of folks. However, the techniques needed to appreciate autostereograms are exactly the ones needed for successful scrying. By attempting to look through the chosen medium, we allow ourselves to disconnect from our rational minds and connect with an older part of our psyche.

Relax. First, focus your eyes gently and then soften your gaze. Allow what you see to become fuzzy. Look through your medium and let your mind wander. Simply acknowledge your thoughts, as they come to you, and then let them pass by, like a drop of water in a gently flowing stream. Once you stop trying to force the visions to come, you will see the images more readily.

You can gaze into any of a number of things: a bowl of salt, a favorite crystal, or the flame of a single candle. Specific examples and techniques follow.

WATER SCRYING

A bowl of water is probably the easiest tool for scrying purposes, as it does not require any special materials. A dark-colored bowl will work best, and it may be helpful to place a drop or two of oil on the surface of the water to give your eye something to focus on at first.

The essential oil of your choice would be helpful here. For example, essential oil of frankincense would ground and center your focus because of its dark resinous smell and its association with religious observances. Studies have also shown frankincense to be an antidepressant. A light, crisp citrus scent like lime would raise your consciousness and clear away the mental cobwebs to bring you to a higher state of being. One drop of essential oil will be plenty for this use. Remember, the oil will float on the water, so don't put too much on the water or your eyes will protect themselves by starting to burn and water.

AIR SCRYING

Air scrying is naturally meditative because swirling incense smoke is inherently hypnotic. It allows your subconscious mind to wander. Nephelomancy, or divination with cloud shapes, is another form of air scrying. Something that I can do only a few times a year where I live is scrying with snowflakes. Watching snow fall, swirl on a breeze, and then land is so relaxing. The thick mass of the snow deadens all sound and lends itself to creating the space for divination. Remember, the method is not the most important thing, as long as you are receiving messages.

What makes scrying such an easy skill to master is that the shapes and visions you see all derive from within your own mind. Therefore, you are the best person to interpret what you see. Your interpretation of a porcupine could be completely different from someone else's. Perhaps you were poked by one as a child, so now you fear them. Meanwhile, your best friend thinks porcupines are cuddly and adorable. You may interpret a porcupine as danger while your friend sees it as indicating a need for therapeutic play.

FIRE SCRYING

Fire scrying can employ a single candle flame or multiple candles. The darker the room at the onset of the meditation, the easier the session. The candle flame will have less light to compete with for your attention. If you experience sensitivity to light, start with a shorter wick and a darkly colored candle to absorb excess light. While unfocusing the eyes, look through the candle flame to the other side while allowing images to form in the mind.

EARTH SCRYING

Earth scrying uses soil, sand, stones, salt, or other earthly media as the visual surface. The practice can be still, or a moving meditation. A prime example would be using a wooden bowl half filled with sand. Placing your hands into the sand to connect with the earth, start sifting your fingers through the sand as well as feeling the sand drift back into the bowl while allowing the mind to drift and muse on the question at hand.

Tea Leaf Reading

Tea leaf reading, or tasseomancy, appears in many books and movies, for example in the Harry Potter series. The difference between tea leaf reading and scrying of any type is that the shapes are easily seen, but understanding them takes practice. Loose-leaf tea, water, and a cup and saucer are the basic supplies needed. Perhaps you would like to invite a friend over for tea to practice reading for each other. Choose a quality tea with a pleasant smell for the best effect. For a traditionally sized teacup, 1 to 1.5 teaspoons of tea is best. Pour your hot water over the tea leaves and allow them to steep for three to five minutes. Chat about your day, work, friends, and anything else you like while sipping your tea. *Do not filter the tea leaves from the cup*. Drinking tea through your teeth may sound awkward, but the tea leaves are the reason you are doing this. Drink until there is only about a tablespoon or two of tea left at the bottom of the cup, Then place the saucer over the top of the cup with a napkin, swirl a few times, and turn the cup over. The napkin in the saucer will absorb any remaining tea, and when you gaze into the teacup you will be able to discern shapes. The shapes closest to you are happening soonest; those shapes farthest away from you are generally interpreted as happening later—perhaps even a year away. Shapes like canoes or boats are interpreted as travel, while X does not mark the spot; this shape is seen as a bad omen. Practice interpreting symbols that come up and assigning meanings. Remember, you are the interpreter here. (See the section on Making Your Own Oracle for interpreting symbols).

Pendulums

Pendulums, or bobs, commonly are made of wood, stone, glass, and metals, among other materials. They may be customized and used in various ways, from locating lost items to dowsing for water. A pendulum is a visual guide to our feelings using our idiomotor reflex.

Because the person holding the pendulum ultimately provides the movement does not mean information received is false or tainted. The bob is controlled by idiopathic movements. The person holding it is moving it, but the movements are subconscious and not controlled.

The easiest way to use a pendulum is to work with it. Yes, really. Hold one end with the index finger and thumb of your dominant hand. With your nondominant hand, hold the bob next to the other end. Ask the pendulum to show you what "yes" looks like and drop the bob end. Watch it swing freely from your dominant hand and note the direction. Does it swing back and forth, or in a circle? Repeat this for "no." It will move in a number of ways. For example, my "yes" looks like a back-and-forth motion in a straight line. My "no" is the circle mimicking the "O" in *no*. If the pendulum drops and quivers, it is a nonanswer. The materials are yours to create. If you love stones, have a stone pendulum for each beloved stone. If you are a woodworker, maybe you can carve bobs out of your favorite wood. The sky is the limit.

ORGANIC PENDULUMS

Health divination can be done by piercing a clove of fresh garlic with a needle strung with red thread and tying off one end. Ask the pendulum health-related questions. For example, "Is Bob on the mend from his bout with the flu?" A similar pendulum can be made with a fresh rosebud for asking love-related questions. Those with fertility or protection questions can use a pinecone.

Bibliomancy

Being an unabashed bibliophile, I love bibliomancy. Grab the book nearest you and open that puppy up! Some purists keep a Bible on hand, because that is how it used to be done. When I remind them that was simply because the book was the most common from house to house, the lightbulb goes on. I prefer fiction books for this. Ask a question, open the book, and pick a sentence with your finger.

Palmistry

Palmistry studies the lines on the hand, their relationships to each other and the mounds, as well as the shapes of the hand and fingers. There are very general things to be learned by concentrating on a single line, like the life line. It can be determined if there was a difficult birth. For example, the start of my life line is a mess of hatch marks. The length of a life line is important as well, but divining the meaning in loops, whirls, broken lines, and other marks is an art. The encyclopedias of palmistry are many; it takes dedication to learn the art, just like other types of divination. Keep in mind that the lines of the hands will deepen and change over time, too. No one's future is set in stone.

Stone Oracles

The easiest stone oracle was suggested by my first high priestess. Place six tumbled clear quartz stones in a bag with six tumbled black tourmaline stones of similar size and weight. This is your yes/no oracle. Next time you have a burning question, draw a stone for an answer (or do two out of three if you are feeling stubborn). Melody's *Love Is in the Earth* is one of the best books for stones, but there are plenty out there. For beginners I also suggest a field guide that breaks the stones up by color, so you can look up stones you find in metaphysical shops once you get them home and have forgotten the name of the stone you just bought.

Making Your Own Oracle

So why am I telling you so much about divination in a book so largely focused on aromatherapy? Because it's all about that inner journey. We are moving together to help you learn more about yourself, where you have been, and where you are going. I'm just piloting the boat; you are charting the course.

There are many kinds of nature oracles you can make with a little time, your imagination, and a few materials. In this section, we'll cover a few different types of oracles you can create for yourself:

↎ Gather fresh flowers from the garden, the grocery store, or your local florist and press them between the pages of a heavy book. Once dried, affix the flowers to card stock to create a flower oracle.

↎ If you're inclined toward illustrations, printing out pictures of flowers and plants (or drawing your own) can be just the ticket for a botanical drawing oracle.

↎ With most cell phones now having incredible cameras built in, why not venture out into the world to take some pictures of local flowers and plants native to where you are? Take as many or as few photos as you would like for your own floral-photo oracle. You can group them into a major and minor arcana like the tarot, or simply find flowers and plants that resonate with you.

↎ Finally, you can learn to interpret the proximity of plants and flowers to your home and work, and detect natural omens. For example, pokeweed can be an insidious plant in the garden. Its purple berries stain clothes and are poisonous to children. But what is poison anyway, but a defense mechanism? We'll learn how to make a potent protection ink out of pokeweed.

Creating a Pressed-Flower Oracle

I found my first pressed flowers (flowers dried in a special press so they can be matted and framed) between the pages of the family Bible when I was a child. Pressed flower kits may be purchased at craft stores and online shops. My first one was the size of a hardback book with brass hardware. I was recently given a larger wooden one that looks like an old-style printing press. It's crucial to use suitable flowers for this process. Succulents and delicate flowers such as petunias, impatiens, and begonias will not work.

If you garden, this is a great way to preserve the bounty of the season. Alternatively, your local craft store should have a delightful selection of dried flowers. Ideally, you'd gather flowers from your own yard, or your friendly neighbors' yards (with permission, of course). Do not take flowers from public gardens without permission, for lots of reasons: the plants might be study specimens; they might recently have been sprayed with toxic chemicals; or it just might simply not be allowed. If someone finds you sneaking through their bushes at night, there is no telling what could happen. It is not worth getting arrested for trespassing, or worse.

If you venture into the woods, make sure you know what you are seeking and can recognize it. Protected species will not be marked. It is your responsibility to know what is legal or illegal to pick. Make sure someone knows where you are going and when to expect you to return. Safety first!

Here's the basic process: Place the flowers between acid-free paper and press it between the pages of a book, or between sheets of cardboard in a press. Leave it there for a few weeks. Mount the dried flowers on card stock and laminate if possible—they will last much longer that way. Low-temperature lamination is the best here to preserve the color of the petals. Dried flowers have a delicate, antique feel to me, so I love working with cards made with this method.

METHOD A

Once you have collected all of your flowers, remove them from their stems and place them into a bowl. It can be wooden or glass, common or unique. Ask for blessings in the manner appropriate to you.

Cast the flowers onto a workspace such as a cotton cloth to keep the flowers in a readable order so you can interpret their shapes. Are many of the flowers face-down? Do any shapes or patterns jump out at you? This is a deeply personal process. I cannot tell you what these shapes mean to you—you must divine that for yourself—but I can give you some general ideas.

Symbols of Misfortune	Symbols of Good Fortune
Crosses or Xs	Crescent Moon
Shovels	Clover
Snakes	Leaves/Flowers
Cats	Fruit
Toads	Circles and Stars

METHOD B

Once you have collected all of your flowers, remove the petals from their buds or stems and place them into a bowl. Ask for blessings in the manner appropriate to your spiritual path. Cast them onto a workspace and interpret their shapes. If you're working with loose petals, it may be easier to divine shapes rather than working with whole flowers, just like with tea leaves. Use the same chart above to give you an idea of the shapes you're looking for.

Creating a Botanical Drawing Oracle

In an age where all the botanical drawings of the world are just a Google image search away, there is still room for the artistic among us to draw or paint our own nature oracle. Your local library will have artist renderings, books on plant life, and field guides to flora and fauna the world over. If you're inclined toward drawing, print-ing out pictures of flowers and plants (or drawing your own) can be just the ticket. Affix the images to cards to create your own personal oracle deck.

Drawing, coloring, and creating art of any kind has been found to be therapeutic, almost as a moving meditation. What better devo-tional than creating your own work of art with self-discovery in mind? You can study the classics from *Culpeper's Complete Herbal*;

it was created in 1653 and is still in print to this day. Other helpful books include Matthew Wood's *The Earthwise Herbal* and Maud Grieve's two-volume set, *A Modern Herbal*.

Creating a Floral-Photo Oracle

Start by going out and taking as many floral, herbal, or plant photos as possible. Most phones come with pretty spectacular cameras in them. If this is your only access to photo-taking, use it.

Once you have a good crop of photos, the weeding process can begin. Start by taking out photos that are blurry, shaky, or out of focus. Once you have taken the time to make a first pass on the group, start assigning meaning to the photos you are left with. None of these methods are about being the most artistic person on the planet. Really. We are trying to tell your subconscious mind the meaning of the photo you have chosen. You may be able to read someone's entire life story from two garden photos. This is your oracle. No one else needs to understand it.

COLORS

The colors of the flowers you choose have significance, and they can have a variety of meanings. A pale pink flower, for example, could mean innocent, romantic love, whereas a bright, fiery red flower could mean anger or passion. Below are some common color correspondences to consider when assigning meaning to your oracle cards.

Color	Meaning
Red	Anger, fire, passion, sexuality
Orange	Part red, part yellow; action of red, intellect of yellow. Business success, abundance
Yellow	Air, intellect, knowledge, good cheer
Green	Earth, fertility, growth, prosperity, balance
Blue	Water, devotion, peace, tranquility, protection
Violet	Spirit, intuition, spirituality, inspiration

NUMBERS

Numbers often display patterns or symbols that may not be recognized right away. Let's take a look at what those numbers might signify.

Number of Flowers	Meaning
1	I love you; you are the one for me
2	Pairs, joining, balance
3	Creation
4	Stability
5	Intensity, passion, Venus
6	Growing love
12	Be mine
24	I belong to you

Going by our charts, a photo of three pale pink roses could be the creation of romantic love, or a new love relationship.

PERSPECTIVE AND COMPOSITION

Perspective in the photos can also be a vital tool. In my original oracle creation, one of the photos I took did not come out as expected. I intended to get a photo of a single rosebud. Instead, what appeared in the review was a photo of some spectacular red roses in the background, and a very blurry single bud in the foreground. Instead of scrapping this photo because it was not the flower I intended, I kept it. This photo was renamed "Perspective" and signifies that the querent does not have a clear view of the problem at hand, or rather "can't see the forest for the trees."

Geographic items can also be featured in your nature oracle. Is the tower in your local park also the Tower card from the tarot? Is it simply a garden oasis in a storm of chaos? A swing set could remind you to stay flexible in your approach to a problem. Keep in mind the areas surrounding the plants and flowers, and these can inform your cards' meanings as well.

SCENT

For a number of years, I worked at a British essential oil–based, fresh, handmade cosmetics company, LUSH, educating folks about essential oils in cosmetics. You would be surprised at the number of people whose entire scent vocabulary consists of oatmeal, Play-Doh, and flowers. By getting out in the world to create a nature oracle, you'll get to know the world around you and increase your scent vocabulary.

Many books discuss visualization and seeing outcomes in your mind's eye, but how many times have you tried to "visualize" a scent? Can you smell things in your mind, like the scent of a freshly peeled orange, or a warm summer night from childhood? Do you have a Rolodex in your mind of the scents you have encountered, or merely a scribbled sticky note hastily stuck to the back of your brain?

There are many meanings for flowers that are encountered in our day-to-day lives. These encounters are largely dismissed, usually due to time constraints. By stopping to smell the roses, or lilacs, or even dandelions, we can start assigning those flowers a scent value in our minds. Remember, we are building a scent vocabulary while designing the nature oracle. On the other hand, some flowers you will encounter do not smell good at all. There is a flower that has gotten national attention in the last few years because of its smell, and that's the corpse flower, *Amorphophallus titanum*. This flower has an impressive stature: a single bud can be over six feet tall. It gets its name and reputation from the scent it gives off. Instead of a rosy glow, or the powdery scent of mums, it smells like rotting meat. So as often as we think of "flowery" as its own scent, remember each plant really has an entire theme all its own.

Then there are flowers with no scent at all. This does not mean they have no value in our nature oracle; it simply means that they are visually enjoyable but will not lend their scent to our endeavors. Fuchsia is one such flower. Its name means "faithfulness," and its delightful tutu-like shape makes it very pleasant to grow and enjoy. Its lack of scent is no detriment to the joy it brings.

TYPE

The types of flowers you choose to photograph are also significant. Below are a handful of meanings for flowers you may come across in your outings.

Flower Type	Meaning
Lantana	Rigor, rigidity, tradition
Bleeding Heart	Undying love
Lilac	Spiritual protection
Thistle	Healing, strength, protection
Bird of Paradise	Unexpected events
Daisy	Innocence
Jasmine	Wealth, elegance

Thistle is one example: the fact that the leaves look sharp is a good reminder that they are good protective flowers. If we used a photo of thistle in our oracle, it could represent a need for protection or that the querent (the person being read) is protected. If the card is reversed, that could mean that there are holes in the querent's defenses.

There are many, many guides that can help determine the meaning of plants and flowers local to you.

Unidentified Plants

Even if you are not sure what the plant in your photo is, it can have meaning. Flowering vines could mean support, help from unknown sources, or even divine intervention. Foliage plants or plants that have yet to flower can read differently than a plant in full bloom. Remember, any plant that can protect itself (usually with thorns, briars, poisons, toxins, or even an itchy rash) can also protect you in the energetic world. Just use caution when touching any plant you don't recognize.

Identifying Omens, Proximity of Flowers and Plants

The proximity of plants and flowers around you can be interpreted. This method is more of a walking meditation on your question. Find a place to start your journey and ask the question needed. Once your question has been established, start walking and interpret what you see.

For example, say you are living in the city and you have a question about whether your current relationship will last. Upon walking out your front door, you see a lone dandelion growing from a crack in the sidewalk. How would you interpret this? Would it remind you to hold on tightly? Would it provide hope in a bleak time? Or does this remind you that you are strong enough to go it alone? Later in your walk, you see a community garden being planted. Does this mean you will reap the rewards of a job well done, or that it is time to sow your seeds elsewhere?

"DANGEROUS" FLOWERS

Not all flowers are nice. For example, poison ivy has flowers. They are actually very small, white flowers with yellow centers. Poisonous flowers can mean caution, careful what you wish for, or things are not what they seem. Keep in mind that the foliage could be interpreted differently from the flowers. Spotting poison ivy flowers near your home or work could represent the need to put on a brave face, while the red leaves of late fall poison ivy could mean danger, do not proceed.

Here's another example: pokeweed can be an insidious plant in the garden. Its purple berries stain clothes, shoes, and the dog's paws. Children are cautioned not to eat the berries because they are poisonous. But those same berries make a potent ink for writing protection spells. If your house is suddenly ringed in a fence of pokeweed, perhaps this means you or your household are in need of protection.

Poke Ink

A young poke (*Phytolacca americana*) plant is succulent and green, but a mature plant has red and purple veins and warns of the toxins inside. Juice from the pokeberry makes a lovely purple ink that can be used to write protection spells or intentions. Having a spat with a neighbor? Write about it with your poke ink. Child going on their first date? Write their name on a piece of paper with your poke ink and place it with a candle until they are home safely.

The thing I like about poke ink protections is that the ink does not last forever. The worries I write disappear over time—just like my poke ink. The pioneers had a recipe that was very easy, and there are plenty of recipes on the internet.

Here's my version:

½ teaspoon vinegar

½ teaspoon salt

¾ cup ripe poke berries

Add the vinegar and salt to a glass bottle. Place the berries in a sealed heavy-duty baggie and mash them with a mortar and pestle. Then strain the seeds and skins and throw them away. The poke seeds are really toxic, so make sure they're disposed of carefully and no one eats them. Add the pokeberry juice to the bottle with the salt and vinegar. It will not last long, so make small batches of ink as needed.

For homemade poke ink, I use a glass pen, rather than a fountain pen. In the off-season, I will add a few drops of my poke ink to a jar of premade ink so it will still have the protective mojo I want when I am not able to get my hands on fresh berries.

Appendices

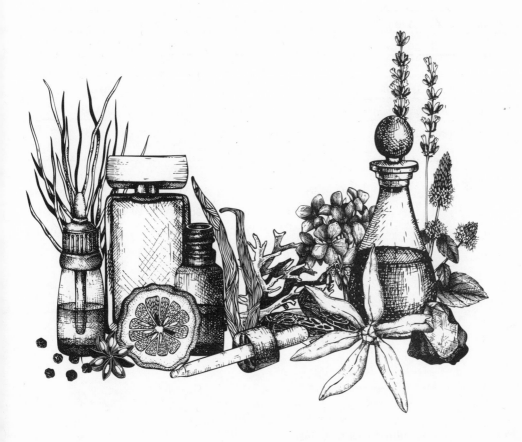

APPENDIX A:
PHOTOTOXICITY AND PROTECTING YOUR SKIN

Some essential oils are phototoxic, meaning that they can cause burns or blisters if they come in contact with skin and direct sunlight and/or UV light from artificial sources. Caution should be used when dealing with these oils and in cases where an alternative is available, it should be investigated.

Essential Oil	Distilled	Expressed
Angelica (*Angelica archangelica*)	Phototoxic	Phototoxic
Bergamot (*Citrus bergamia*)	Non-phototoxic	Phototoxic
Bitter Orange (*Citrus aurantium*)	Non-phototoxic	Phototoxic
Grapefruit (*Citrus paradisi*)	Non-phototoxic	Small concern
Lemon (*Citrus limon*)	Non-phototoxic	Phototoxic
Persian Lime (*Citrus latifolia*)	Non-phototoxic	Phototoxic
Myrrh (*Commiphora myrrha*)	Phototoxic	Phototoxic
Neroli (*Citrus aurantium*)	Non-phototoxic	Non-phototoxic
Sweet Orange (*Citrus sinensis*)	Non-phototoxic	Non-phototoxic
Petitgrain (*Citrus aurantium*)	Non-phototoxic	Non-phototoxic
Tangerine/Mandarin (*Citrus reticulate*)	Non-phototoxic	Non-phototoxic

Avoid direct sunlight after exposure to these oils for twelve to seventy-two hours, depending on the sensitivity of the skin. In cases where sunlight exposure cannot be avoided, apply to areas covered by clothing or apply the oil or synergy to an aroma locket or on a tissue inside a pocket.

APPENDIX B:
OILS TO AVOID DURING PREGNANCY

Note: This is not a complete list. Consult with a doctor, midwife, trained aromatherapist, or herbalist before using essential oils while pregnant.

Essential Oil	Latin Name
Aniseed	*Pimpinella anisum*
Anise, Star	*Illicium verum*
Basil	*Ocimum basilicum*
Birch	*Betula lenta*
Blue Cypress	*Callitris intratropica*
Camphor	*Cinnamomum camphora*
Chamomile (Roman)	*Chamaemelum nobile*
Clary Sage	*Salvia sclarea*
Fennel, Sweet	*Foeniculum vulgare*
Ho leaf	*Cinnamomum camphora*
Hyssop	*Hyssopus officinalis*
Mugwort	*Artemisia vulgaris*
Myrtle	*Myrtus communis*
Nutmeg	*Myristica fragrans*
Parsley	*Petroselinum sativum*
Pennyroyal	*Mentha pulegium*
Rosemary	*Rosmarinus officinalis*
Sage	*Salvia officinalis*
Spanish lavender	*Lavandula stoechas*
Spearmint	*Mentha spicata*
Tarragon	*Artemisia dracunculus*
Wintergreen	*Gaultheria procumbens*

If exposure to essential oils results in drops contacting sensitive mucus membranes (e.g., in the nose) or splashes into eyes, flush with full-fat milk or a few drops of jojoba oil.

APPENDIX C:
TESTING YOUR ESSENTIAL OILS FOR QUALITY AND PURITY

The quality and purity of essential oils can vary widely, and some companies dilute their product more than others. But there are things you can do: perform essential oil integrity tests, ask the manufacturer for more information, and do your own side-by-side comparisons of different brands.

It is most important to test the following kinds of oils:

- *Any oil that uses the word "pure," "natural," "premium," "certified," or "therapeutic grade" on its label.* There is no such thing as a governing body that certifies or grades essential oil. These are marketing terms. The tiny ™ next to that phrase means it is a trademarked term and means nothing for purity.

- *Any essential oil derived from a resin.* It is common to dilute a resin-based oil with water, chemicals, or other oils and not list it on the label, and still charge outrageous prices.

- *Any oil listed as an absolute (e.g., jasmine, neroli, oakmoss, vanilla, and rose).* The more expensive an oil is, the less likely it has been adulterated. (Do not take this for granted, though. Still test your expensive oils to confirm quality.) True absolutes are thick and difficult to work with, and may require a water bath to work with; see Oakmoss for details.

Dead giveaways your oils have been adulterated:

- *Any oil sold in a clear glass container.* Clear glass lets all the ultraviolet light into the bottle and can degrade the quality of the oil within rapidly.

- *All the oils in a supplier's line having the same price.* Every essential oil needs a different amount of plant material to create the product, and materials are obtained from all over the world. If the price of rose oil is the same as lavender, something is off.

- *Extra-large bottles of expensive oils selling at surprisingly low prices.* Large bottles of some oils are common—for example, peppermint or lavender essential oil will be relatively inexpensive. If a hard-to-obtain oil is being sold in a large container outside of a commercial application, it should be suspect. Synthetics have their use and enjoyment but pose no benefit for the purposes of magical aromatherapy. In the realm of magic, the natural world is in play.

- *Color and viscosity seem inconsistent with other brands.* Resins, grasses, and other oils should be darker and more viscous than essential oils derived from flowers and leaves.

TESTING METHODS

These methods will save you time and money and potentially avoid health hazards like allergy-related cross contamination.

Evidence of Water Dilution

Add a few tablespoons of water to a glass and stir. Notice how plain water returns to its natural state within a second or so, no matter how hard it is stirred or for how long. Place a drop of essential oil in the water, and stir. If the oil is unadulterated, there might be a slight film but the water will still look mostly like water. If large globules of oil are visible, it is likely the oil was diluted with a carrier oil, like jojoba. If the water turns thick and cloudy, with many bubbles on the surface, the oil has been diluted with water and mixed with an emulsifier to get the oil and water to blend.

Evidence of Oil Dilution

Draw a circle or square on a sheet paper. Underneath list the following:

- Current date and time
- Brand of essential oil to be tested
- Oil's common name
- Oil's Latin binomial
- Oil's batch number, if there is one

Place 1 drop of essential oil inside the shape. Note the color, scent, viscosity, and other notable characteristics.

Wait one hour, and check the drop again. Notice the oil's scent, color, and staining. The scent will have dissipated in some of the lighter oils, such as citrus oils. Depending on whether the oil was steam distilled or expressed, there may be color staining the circle. With a true essential oil, the paper will wrinkle, as though the spot is a drop of water. If the paper shows large, greasy spots, the oil has been diluted with carrier oil. If the label does not state the oil was diluted, there is an issue.

Check the drop again twenty-four hours later. The more viscous the oil, the longer the scent will last. The scent should be faint for middle notes and completely gone for top notes. If you are testing a base note the scent may still be identifiable for forty-eight hours after application.

If the smell is still going as strong after two or three days, it is either a fragrance oil or heavily adulterated.

Other Methods for Assessing Oil Quality

EXPERIENCE

Oftentimes the best teacher is experience. If Brand A consistently shows signs of mixing water and emulsifiers with their oils, buy from another company. Many stores that sell essential oils have testers that are open and can be smelled or tested before buying. Take them up on it.

LOCATION

The closer the plant material production site is to its native habitat, the more likely the essential oil is to be pure. This is not a guarantee, but it's helpful to consider.

ORGANIC/WILD CRAFTED

While words like "pure" and "true" have no meaning outside marketing for essential oils, the word "organic" does. For an essential oil to be labeled "organic," it has to hold up to a rigorous standard. Organic farms are susceptible to surprise inspections of their property, soil, and equipment. Another term you might see on labels is "wild crafted." This means that the plant materials were gathered in the wild, rather than farmed, and the term carries with it connotations of biodiversity, all-natural ingredients (no chemicals), and earth stewardship.

SMELL

It seems overly simple, but our sense of smell is our greatest asset. The variances in scent will be more noticeable if the original oil is at hand. Scents of jojoba or other carriers will also be more noticeable.

GCMS DATA SHEETS

See if the manufacturer can provide GCMS (gas chromatography/mass spectroscopy) data sheets for the oils it produces. Having this data shows the company takes its oils and production methods seriously, but the report won't spell out everything for you. Here are a few ways oils can be adulterated that will not show up on a GCMS test:

- A better-quality batch of essential oil may be mixed with a lower-quality oil of the same genus and species and it will still show as a true essential oil (just as cheap gas stations may add things to gasoline that will lower the quality without affecting the octane rating).

- A cheaper essential oil with a similar chemical makeup may be added to the "true" oil.

- A company may add natural components or synthetic versions of the oil.

- Oils may be heated to burn off undesirable scents.

- A GCMS test cannot determine if an essential oil has been distilled more than once to concentrate volatile oils.

APPENDIX D:
BOTANICAL MAGIC RESOURCES

At the time of this printing, these companies were known to produce quality, ethically sourced materials. No payment was received by the author for mention in these pages.

Twilight Alchemy Lab is, according to its website, "the fruit of a millennia of research, hands-on experimentation and investigation in the history, theory and practice of alchemy, the Hermetic Sciences, the art of rootwork and aromatherapy as it pertains to ritual, spirituality and low magick." *twilightalchemylab.com*

Black Phoenix Alchemy Lab, an esoteric perfume house based in North Hollywood, California, produces dragon's blood perfume of the highest quality. I highly recommend them. *blackphoenixalchemylab.com*

Got Oil Supplies offers a wide variety of bottle sizes for blending. *gotoilsupplies.com*

Lunaroma essential oils. *lunaroma.com*

Miracle Botanicals, a family-owned farm in Hawaii, grows as much of its material as it can for its essential oils. *miraclebotanicals.com*

Nature's Gift is a good source for buying basic essential oils online. *naturesgift.com*

Piping Rock is a good source for both basic essential oils and harder-to-find materials, like oakmoss. *pipingrock.com*

Specialty Bottle offers containers of all sizes, shapes, and colors. *specialtybottle.com*

Stillpoint Aromatics essential oils. *stillpointaromatics.com*

If you want to learn more about aromatics, check out the accredited New York Institute of Aromatic Studies. *aromaticstudies.com*

Glossary of Botanical Magic Terms

A

absolute   Oil procured via solvent extraction, rather than steam distillation. This extra step creates a rich and full-bodied oil, but is often a bit more expensive. Delicate materials such as jasmine, neroli, oakmoss, and rose that would be damaged by heat or pressure are commonly solvent extracted.

altar   A flat space used for sacred items, ritual tools, and candles used for prayer, meditation, intention work, and spells. Can be permanent or temporary.

amulet   A magical token; a symbol of a magical working. Pendants, rings, necklaces, and other types of jewelry are common amulets. The difference is being blessed or consecrated to a specific task. *See also: talisman.*

aromatherapy   The art and science of using true botanical essences to create change in the mind, body, and spirit of individuals or groups through scent. Not all smells are aromatherapy; this is a marketing technique. To have therapeutic benefit beyond a pleasant smell, essential oils must be used.

athame (ATH-a-may)   A double-edged ritual dagger used to direct energy and cast a circle. Not used for cutting physical items. (For cutting herbs and other physical items, see *boline*.)

aura   The invisible energy field that surrounds all living things.

B

banish   To drive away energies.

bind   To restrict the energy or intentions of another. Commonly, to prevent harm.

binomial   The two-part scientific name of a plant. These two parts refer to the genus and species. These names are incredibly important in that different members of the same family can act in different ways, have separate effects on the body, and can cause allergic reactions between species. For example, one could have an allergic reaction to Turkish rose (*Rosa damascena*) while having no allergic symptoms to the English rose (*Rosa centifolia*).

blend   For the purposes of this book, the word blend refers largely to two or more essential oils diluted in a carrier.

boline (BOW-leen)   Crescent-shaped ritual knife used to harvest herbs for workings, medicines, teas, and other uses. Frequently white-handled.

Book of Shadows   The diary of a tradition of a witch, or workings performed and results attained. In traditional witchcraft, the shadow was not "bad"; it was merely the Trap Street, or fictitious entry of the witch. Each group chooses something to write down in their book that they know is incorrect so that if someone copies their book, they know it was stolen from their group. (A witch may have more than one Book of Shadows.) *See also grimoire.*

botanical   Of or pertaining to botany, the science of plants.

C

carrier oil   Fat-based oil (usually from nuts and seeds) that allows for the integration of essential oils without an emulsifier. Because applying undiluted essential oils directly to the skin causes burning and irritation, a carrier oil allows even distribution and absorption by the skin. Common carrier oils include coconut, jojoba, coconut, olive, sunflower seed, and sweet almond.

censer   Vessel or fireproof dish, often brass, used for burning incense.

centering   Taking all of one's scattered energy and concentrating it in the center of the physical body, calming.

chakra   Energy centers in the body. Traditionally, there are seven (root, sacral, solar plexus, heart, throat, third eye, and crown), though more are recognized.

charm   A magical tool aimed at a specific goal. For example, a white muslin bag filled with cedarwood, lavender buds, and amethyst could be used as a charm to cleanse and calm the mind.

chemotype   Essential oils of the same variety, for example thyme (*Thymus vulgaris*), where the growing habit, soil composition, and altitude affect the chemical composition. These oils will have a separate designation (ct) along with their name, such as thyme, linalol (*Thymus vulgaris ct linalol*). Separate chemotypes will have different uses. This is not the same as hybridization (e.g., lavendin vs. lavender), as the plants still share the same Latin binomial. Other such essential oils that offer chemotypes are chamomile, eucalyptus, and salvia.

consecration   Blessing; imbuing an object with sacred, protective, or holy energy.

D

diffuser   A device that disperses essential oil into the air. These can be electric appliances that disperse water vapor with essential oils diluted within for therapeutic and aromatic benefit. An aroma locket or salt can also be utilized; simply empty a few drops of essential oil into a few tablespoons of salt, stir well, and leave out.

divination   A means of deciphering events outside of normal perception. Examples include dreaming, tarot, scrying, oracle cards, and runes.

dram   A unit of measure equivalent to one eighth of a fluid ounce.

E

esbat   A witch's worship time, with or without other participants, usually held on the new or full moon.

essential oil   The main product of the distillation of plant-based materials used for the therapeutic benefit of the physical, the mental, and, for the purposes of this book, the magical.

F

fixative   An essential oil that is more viscous and will extend the scent of the perfume on the skin, or in the air, "fixing" it.

G

grimoire   The recipe book of a witch, which may contain instructions and recipes for ointments, oils, and more. A Book of Shadows can be the witch's personal journey, the grimoire the cookbook.

ground   To anchor oneself to the physical world—a very calming and nurturing practice.

H

hydrosol The by-product of steam distillation of materials for essential oil production. The oil is lighter than the water and is drained off. The remaining water contains .02 to .03 percent dissolved oil in water.

M

magic(k) According to Aleister Crowley, it's "the Art and Science of causing Change to occur in conformity with Will." Occasionally spelled with the letter "k" to differentiate between stage illusions and religious energy work.

morphology The parts of the plants used. Each entry will list the part of the plant where the oil is derived. This serves several purposes. There are essential oils where a single plant is used to make several essential oils of differing names, for example *Citrus aurantium*. Three essential oils are created from this singular tree, the bitter orange. The peel of this member of the citrus family produces bitter orange essential oil. The flowers of the bitter orange tree produce neroli essential oil, and the leaves of the bitter orange tree produce petitgrain essential oil. Each has a slightly different scent; two are top notes, where petitgrain is a delightful middle note. Morphology can also explain why essentials are so vastly different in cost. Melissa, for example, comes from the prolific lemon balm plant, but only the flowering tops are used for essential oil production. Essential oils derived from resins will be more expensive because the trees take two decades to mature enough to produce the sap that will eventually dry to form resin drops called tears.

N

neat Undiluted. The application of an essential oil directly to the skin without carrier oil. Not recommended. Poses a danger to the skin and mucosal membranes and can result in burns, hives, skin sensitization, and other health hazards. The only essential oil found to safely be used neat is lavender (*Lavandula angustifolia*), and while generally regarded as safe, it has its limitations as well. (Lavender should be avoided by pregnant women unless under the careful supervision and treatment by a certified aromatherapist, as miscarriages can occur.)

note   An isolated scent in a blended fragrance (e.g., a note of jasmine). Top notes evaporate the fastest and will be smelled first in a blend. Middle notes give the top notes a bit of staying power, but are still moving at a stately pace. Base notes last the longest in perfumes and on the skin.

P

pentacle   A physical object showing a five-pointed star in a circle called a pentagram. Often placed on an altar for consecrating tools, oils, or charms. A single point up represents humans reaching out to the Universe, for something outside themselves. Two points up is often indicative of the second degree in traditional witchcraft and the witch journeying inward in self-discovery. Nothing negative is implied by either positioning.

pentagram   A two-dimensional symbol depicting a five-pointed star in a circle. The five points represent earth, air, fire, water, and spirit.

R

rede   Advice or counsel, not law or commandment. Example: The Wiccan Rede, "Eight words the Wiccan Rede fulfill, 'An harm ye none, do what you will.'" This is not a commandment, but rather counsel to treat others in a manner you would wish to be treated, similar to the Golden Rule.

ritual   Observance, religious or otherwise. A spell can be a part of a larger ceremonial framework involving liturgy, specific actions, and participants.

S

scry   A type of divination involving meditation and trance work, in an attempt to see events in the past, future, or distant places. Scrying in earth, air, fire, and water are common methods.

smudge   The ceremony of Native American and First Nations people of wafting smoldering plant material to cleanse an area of negative energies.

spell   Directed energy and action toward a desired goal. An enacted prayer that can involve candles, chants, dances, or other ritualized action. *See also magic(k)*.

synergy   The amalgamation of two or more essential oils for proscribed use—magical, physical, or emotional. These are primarily designed for diffusing in a water diffuser, storing in an aroma locket, or using in a stick inhaler or salt diffuser.

T

talisman   A magical token; a symbol of a magical working. Pendants, rings, necklaces, and other jewelry are common amulets. The difference is being blessed or consecrated to a specific task.

tear   A single piece of resin, like frankincense, which drips from the plant and resembles tears.

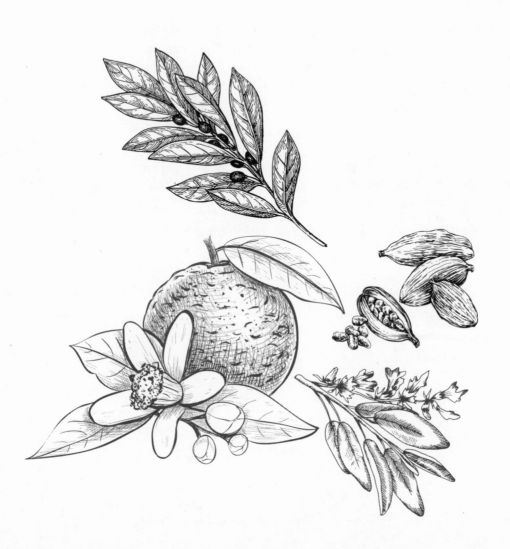

Recipe
Index

BANISHING

Recipe . . . . Essential Oil

Big, Bad Be Gone Oil . . . . Sandalwood

Drive Away Evil . . . . Clove

Ex-Breaking (Banish Ex-Lovers) . . . . Oakmoss

Freedom Spell . . . . Geranium

Happy Trails Oil . . . . Bay

Hex-Breaking Spray . . . . Rosemary

Hex-Removing Bath . . . . Angelica

Hex Shattering . . . . Cedarwood

Incense to Banish Evil . . . . Anise

Multipurpose Banishing Oil . . . . Black Pepper

Obstacle-Removing Diffuser Blend . . . . Bay

Obstacle-Removing Incense . . . . Bay

BLESSING

Recipe . . . . Essential Oil

Baby Blessing . . . . Jasmine

Bless This House Floor Sweep . . . . .Cinnamon

Blessings of the God Diffuser Oil . . . . Angelica

Funeral Blessing Anointing Oil. . . . . Angelica

House Blessing . . . . .Lavender

New Addition Oil . . . . Basil

Time to Leave the Nest. . . . . Bergamot

EMOTIONAL WELL-BEING

Recipe . . . .**Essential Oil**

Anger into Action. . . . . Cardamom

Bodily Acceptance Working . . . . Patchouli

Burnout Biter . . . . Basil

Chill Out, Cheer Up! . . . . .Grapefruit

Choral Bells (Uplifting) . . . . Orange

Comfort Food . . . . .Grapefruit

Count Your Blessings . . . . .Black Pepper

Cupid's Bow. . . . . Clove

Doubt-Be-Gone Empowering Mist. . . . . Bay

Ex-Breaking (Banish Ex Lovers). . . . . Oakmoss

Forgive Yourself. . . . . .Coriander

Forgiveness Massage Oil . . . . Angelica

Frayed Friend Fixer . . . . .Chamomile

Getting to Know You. . . . . Tangerine

Happy Trails Oil . . . . .Bay

Heart Protector . . . . Cardamom

Joy Bath Salts. . . . . Anise

Lady Lust Massage Oil. . . . . .Cinnamon

Lasting Love. . . . . Orange

Love Drawing Bath . . . . Patchouli

Lunar Love. . . . . .Coriander

Magnet Oil. . . . . Lemongrass

Make the First Move . . . . Vetiver

My Mistress's Eyes. . . . . Oakmoss

Ready for Love Anointing Oil . . . . Basil
Strengthen Romantic Relationships . . . . Ginger
To See through Emotions . . . . Ginger
Wedding Night(ly) . . . . Chamomile

HEALING

Recipe . . . . **Essential Oil**
Fruitful Healing . . . . Cinnamon
Healer's Helper . . . . Chamomile
Health and Wellness Soak . . . . Lavender
Recovery . . . . Cedarwood
Self-Improvement . . . . Neroli

MENTAL POWERS

Recipe . . . . **Essential Oil**
Centering Oil . . . . Black Pepper
Clarity Incense . . . . Cardamom
Divination Simmer Potpourri . . . . Anise
Focus-Pocus . . . . Basil
Go, Baby, Go Anointing Oil . . . . Angelica
Into the Dreaming . . . . Nutmeg
Muse Minder . . . . Eucalyptus
Other Realms . . . . Cardamom
Preternatural Prowess . . . . Coriander
Psychic Defender . . . . Cedarwood
Quiet Voices Divination Oil . . . . Lemongrass
Scrying Secrets . . . . Coriander
Steady Ground (Grounding Oil) . . . . Lemongrass

MONEY

Recipe . . . . **Essential Oil**
Bright Business Mojo . . . . Clove
Business Plan Booster . . . . Bergamot

Clean Cash. . . . . Clary Sage
Earthly Delights Prosperity Oil. . . . . .Cedarwood
Here's to Success Cocktail . . . . Bergamot
Luck Luster . . . . .Chamomile
Monetary Do-Over . . . . Basil
Money Honey . . . . Clary Sage
Payment Due . . . . Patchouli
Prosperity Abounds Spell. . . . . Orange
Quick and Dirty Prosperity Spell . . . . Tangerine
Raining Sunshine . . . . Orange

Peace

Recipe . . . . Essential Oil
Calming Communication. . . . . Coriander
Comfort Bath. . . . . Rosemary
Deep Breaths . . . . Lemon
Emotional Balance Oil. . . . . Anise
Garden of Eden . . . . Cardamom
Grounding Anxiety . . . . Patchouli
Harmony Spell. . . . . Orange
Hope Chest Healer. . . . . .Cedarwood
Hypnos Hibernation . . . . Bergamot
Lady Liberty. . . . . Geranium
Let It Go!. . . . . .Chamomile
Letting Go Spell . . . . Geranium
Lift Spirits, Gain Focus Oil. . . . . Vetiver
Lovely Hostess. . . . . Tangerine
Lunar Lady . . . . .Cedarwood
Meditation Oil. . . . . .Lavender
Mercy. . . . . .Myrrh
New Bee. . . . . Eucalyptus
Peaceful Endings . . . . .Peppermint
Rearview Mirror . . . . Ginger

Rosemary Remembrance Tea . . . . Rosemary
Rosewater . . . . Rose
The Seeker . . . . .Black Pepper
Strength of the Goddess Oil . . . . Clove
Tension Tamer Bath Oil . . . . .Neroli
Tough Cookie . . . . Coriander

PROTECTION

Recipe . . . . **Essential Oil**
Anise Protection Incense. . . . . Anise
Battle Hexes. . . . . Lemongrass
Binding, Bending . . . . .Cedarwood
Divine Light Protection Oil . . . . .Lavender
Incoming!. . . . . .Frankincense
Justice . . . . .Jasmine
Kid Gloves Spell. . . . . Rose
Lie Detector . . . . Lemongrass
None Shall Pass . . . . .Frankincense
Protection Garlic Pepper Butter . . . . .Black Pepper
Protective Powder . . . . .Black Pepper
Psychic Protection Cookies. . . . . Anise
Strong Roots . . . . .Cinnamon
True Faces . . . . Cardamom

PURIFICATION

Recipe . . . . **Essential Oil**
All-Purpose Ritual Diffuser Oil . . . . Bay
All-Purpose Ritual Incense . . . . Bay
Energetic Cleansing Floor Wash. . . . . Clove
Florida Water Cologne. . . . . Clove
Home Cleansing Anointing Oil . . . . Angelica
Ritual Tool Consecration Oil . . . . Anise
Sacred Anointing Oil . . . . .Cinnamon

Spring Cleaning . . . . Lemon
Thrice Purified . . . . .Lavender

WORSHIP

Recipe . . . . **Essential Oil**
Beltane Blessings Anointing Oil . . . . .Lavender
Daily Devotional . . . . Geranium
Hallowed . . . . Cardamom
High Priestess Oil. . . . . ∴.Neroli
Imbolc Oil . . . . Angelica
Lammas Leavening. . . . . .Neroli
Litha Lessons . . . . Lemongrass
Long Night's Ritual Work . . . . .Bay
Mabon Memories. . . . . Rosemary
Ostara Dreaming . . . . .Chamomile
Samhain (Faux) Sourdough . . . . Rosemary
Song of the New Wood Initiation Oil. . . . . .Black Pepper
Yule Blessings. . . . . Clove

Bibliography

Beyerl, Paul. *A Compendium of Herbal Magick*. Custer, WA: Phoenix Publishing, 1998.

Blanche, Cynthia. *The Book of Touch & Aroma: Sensual Ways with Massage and Aromatherapy*. Alexandria, VA: Time Life Books, 1997.

Buckland, Raymond. *The Witch Book: The Encyclopedia of Witchcraft, Wicca, and Neo-paganism*. Detroit: Visible Ink Press, 2002.

Chamberlain, Lisa. *Wicca Herbal Magic: A Beginner's Guide to Practicing Wiccan Herbal Magic, with Simple Herb Spells*. N.p.: Wicca Shorts, 2015.

Cunningham, Scott. *Cunningham's Book of Shadows: The Path of an American Traditionalist*. Woodbury, MN: Llewellyn Publications, 2009.

———. *Cunningham's Encyclopedia of Magical Herbs*, 2nd ed. Woodbury, MN: Llewellyn Publications, 2003.

———. *Magical Aromatherapy: The Power of Scent*. St. Paul, MN: Llewellyn Publications, 1997.

Dodt, Colleen K. *The Essential Oils Book: Creating Personal Blends for Mind & Body*. Pownal, VT: Storey Publishing, 1996.

Dubats, Sally. *Natural Magick: Inside the Well-Stocked Witch's Cupboard*. New York: Kensington Books, 1999.

Dugan, Ellen. *Cottage Witchery: Natural Magick for Hearth and Home*. Woodbury, MN: Llewellyn Publications, 2005.

———. *Garden Witch's Herbal: Green Magick, Herbalism & Spirituality*. Woodbury, MN: Llewellyn Publications, 2009.

Essential Oils Desk Reference, 3rd ed. Orem, UT: Essential Science Publishing, 2008.

Fallon, Michael. *Llewellyn's Herbal Almanac*. St. Paul, MN: Llewellyn, 2004.

Franklin, Anna. *The Hearth Witch's Compendium: Magical and Natural Living for Every Day*. Woodbury, MN: Llewellyn, 2017.

Giesecke, Annette. *The Mythology of Plants: Botanical Lore from Ancient Greece and Rome*. Los Angeles: J. Paul Getty Museum, 2014.

Gregg, Susan. *The Complete Illustrated Encyclopedia of Magical Plants*. Beverly, MA: Fair Winds, 2014.

Griggs, Barbara. *Green Pharmacy: The History and Evolution of Western Herbal Medicine*. Rochester, VT: Healing Arts Press, 1997.

Hawkins-Tillirson, Judith. *The Weiser Concise Guide to Herbal Magick*. York Beach, ME: Weiser Books, 2007.

Heath, Maya. *Magical Oils by Moonlight*. Franklin Lakes, NJ: New Page Books, 2004.

Holland, Eileen. *Holland's Grimoire of Magickal Correspondences: A Ritual Handbook*. Franklin Lakes, NJ: New Page Books, 2006.

Illes, Judika. *The Big Book of Practical Spells: Everyday Magic That Works*. Newburyport, MA: Weiser Books, 2016.

Jordan, Michael. *Plants of Mystery and Magic: A Photographic Guide*. New York: Sterling Publishing, 1997.

Keniston-Pond, Kymberly. *Essential Oils 101: Your Guide to Understanding and Using Essential Oils*. Avon, MA: Adams Media, 2017.

Loughran, Joni, and Ruah Bull. *Aromatherapy Anointing Oils: Spiritual Blessings, Ceremonies & Affirmations*. Berkeley, CA: Frog, Ltd., 2001.

Miller, Richard Alan, and Iona Miller. *The Magical and Ritual Use of Perfumes*. Rochester, VT: Destiny Books, 1990.

Morrison, Dorothy. *Everyday Magic: Spells & Rituals for Modern Living*, 1st ed. St. Paul, MN: Llewellyn Publications, 1999.

Murphy-Hiscock, Arin. *The Way of the Hedge Witch: Rituals and Spells for Hearth and Home*. Avon, MA: Provenance Press, 2009.

Perry, Sara. *The Book of Herbal Teas: A Guide to Gathering, Brewing, and Drinking.* San Francisco: Chronicle Books, 1997.

Raven, Hazel. *Heal Yourself with Crystals: Crystal Medicine for Body, Emotions and Spirit.* London: Godsfield, 2005.

RavenWolf, Silver. *Solitary Witch: The Ultimate Book of Shadows for the New Generation,* 1st ed. Woodbury, MN: Llewellyn Publications, 2003.

Telesco, Patricia. *The Victorian Flower Oracle: The Language of Nature.* St. Paul, MN: Llewellyn Publications, 1994.

Tietze, Harald W. *Herbal Teaology.* Bermagui South, NSW, Australia: Harald W. Tietze Publishing, 1996.

Valnet, Jean. *The Practice of Aromatherapy: A Classic Compendium of Plant Medicines & Their Healing Properties.* Rochester, VT: Healing Arts Press, 1990.

West, Kate. *The Real Witches' Garden: Spells, Herbs, Plants and Magical Spaces Outdoors.* Woodbury, MN: Llewellyn Publications, 2004.

Wood, Jamie. *The Wicca Herbal: Recipes, Magick, and Abundance.* Berkeley, CA: Celestial Arts, 2003.

Wood, Matthew. *The Earthwise Herbal: A Complete Guide to Old World Medicinal Plants.* Berkeley, CA: North Atlantic Books, 2008.

Yronwode, Catherine. (2002). *Hoodoo Herb and Root Magic: A Materia Magica of African-American Conjure.* Forestville, CA: Lucky Mojo Curio Company, 2002.

Acknowledgments

A book is never written in a vacuum. Thank you to everyone who has been there loving me, supporting me, named and unnamed. In no particular order: #TAM; Natalie Zaman; my editor, Judika Illes (no turquoise, lol), and everyone at Weiser Books who helped create this book. Heather Grothaus, H. Byron Ballard, Star Bustamonte, Dorothy Morrison, Patti Wigington, experts and talents, all. Thank you, Lord Brian and Whitemarsh Theod. Mama Lori and Mystickal Voyage. JMJ: I love you. Michael: you remind me when I need to hear it; thank you. Amanda: Manhattans in Manhattan, on me. LH: I can't wait for you to hold this book. MK: Dinner on me. Thanks for listening. Kane: deserted island party, taking bets on how long before the rescue crew shows. Kristin: thank you for walking into Brew Ha-Ha. I love you. Caroline K.: thank you for listening. To Miss Mellie, for showing my mother this was never just a phase. To the people who couldn't wait to hold this book. And to you, gentle reader—yes, you.

ABOUT THE AUTHOR

Amy Blackthorn has been described as an "arcane horticulturalist" for her lifelong work with magical plants and teaching of hoodoo and plant-based magic. She incorporates her experiences in British Traditional Witchcraft with her horticulture studies. She is trained as a clinical aromatherapist and is ordained through the Gryphon's Grove School of Shamanism.

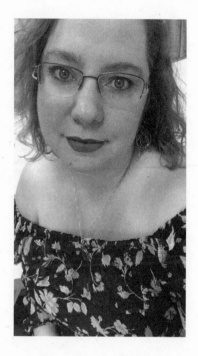

Amy has appeared on *HuffPost Live*, *Yahoo News*, and *Top 10 Secrets and Mysteries* (Episode: "Supernatural Abilities"). Her interviews have appeared in the *Associated Press*, the *Baltimore Sun*, *BankRate.com*, *Realtor.com*, the *Connecticut Post,* and more.

Amy's company, Blackthorn Hoodoo Blends, creates tea based on old Hoodoo formulas. She lives in Delaware.

Visit her at *www.amyblackthorn.com.*

To Our Readers

Weiser Books, an imprint of Red Wheel/Weiser, publishes books across the entire spectrum of occult, esoteric, speculative, and New Age subjects. Our mission is to publish quality books that will make a difference in people's lives without advocating any one particular path or field of study. We value the integrity, originality, and depth of knowledge of our authors.

Our readers are our most important resource, and we appreciate your input, suggestions, and ideas about what you would like to see published.

Visit our website at *www.redwheelweiser.com* to learn about our upcoming books and free downloads, and be sure to go to *www.redwheelweiser.com/newsletter* to sign up for newsletters and exclusive offers.

You can also contact us at *info@rwwbooks.com* or at

Red Wheel/Weiser, LLC
65 Parker Street, Suite 7
Newburyport, MA 01950